Love, Attachment and Intellectual Disability

Meeting Emotional Needs and Developmental Trauma

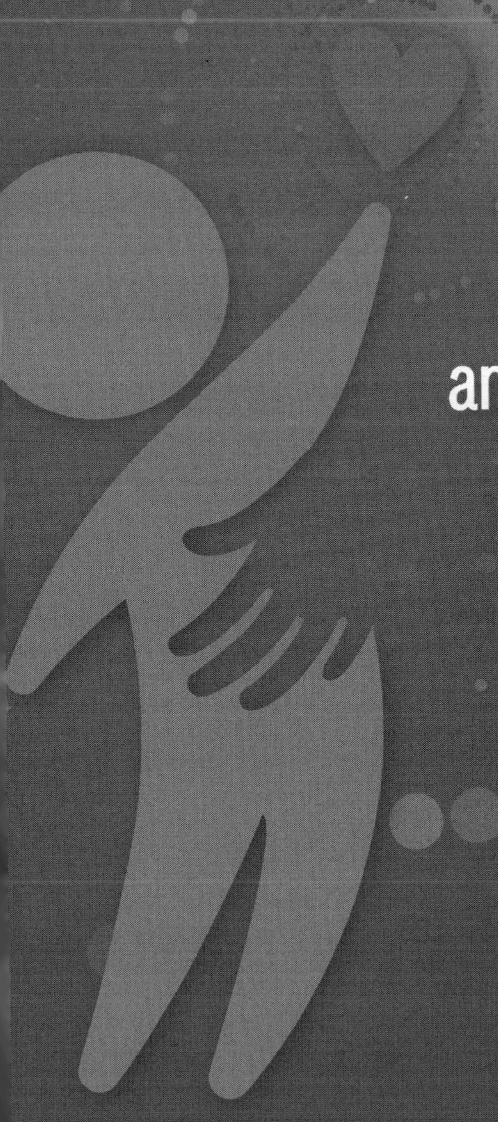

Victoria Shimmens
and Allan Skelly

Pavilion
PUBLISHING

Love, Attachment and Intellectual Disability

Meeting Emotional Needs and Developmental Trauma

Published by:

Pavilion Publishing and Media Ltd
Blue Sky Offices
25 Cecil Pashley Way
Shoreham by Sea
West Sussex
BN43 5FF

Tel: 01273 434 943
Email: info@pavpub.com
Web: www.pavpub.com

Published 2023

A catalogue record for this book is available from the British Library.

ISBN: 978-1-803883-24-3

Pavilion Publishing and Media is a leading publisher of books, training materials and digital content in mental health, social care and allied fields. Pavilion and its imprints offer must-have knowledge and innovative learning solutions underpinned by sound research and professional values.

Authors: Victoria Shimmens and Allan Skelly
Editor: Mike Benge
Cover design: Emma Dawe, Pavilion Publishing and Media Ltd
Page layout and typesetting: Emma Dawe, Pavilion Publishing and Media Ltd
Printing: Independent Publishers Group (IPG)

This book is dedicated to every child,
and the child within every adult.

May they never be without love.

For the Want of Love

I felt your skin
There was too much cold
I looked at you
Few smiles but scolds

My cries unheard
Or just met with shouts
They were there for a time
But now nowhere abouts

I crawled around
All by myself
I was left with those
Who left me with welts

When teacher chided or frowned
I collapsed inside
They bully me for how I look and sound
All self-esteem died

They say I have moods
And should take these wonder pills
They say "challenging behaviour"
And that I should learn more skills

I must be independent
"Resilient", make do
Then hooray the money is saved
For the accountant – that's who

I have "mental illness"
To add to the list
But all of these 'helpers'
The main point they've missed

Not chemicals, brain, genetics nor cell
No none of the above
Truth be told – it was all
For The Want of Love

Anonymous

Contents

"If a community values its children, it must value its mothers."

John Bowlby
Architect of Attachment Theory

*"Not everything that is faced can be changed.
But nothing can be changed until it is faced."*

James Baldwin
Poet, playwright, civil rights activist

*"People need to be kind to children with disabilities.
A little bit more care and protection. Children with disabilities
need a little more. Don't push a little one away when
they're naughty or ask for attention. That's how we get mental
health problems – because we think, 'No one loves me'."*

Roger Wilczek, 2022
Expert by experience

About the authors

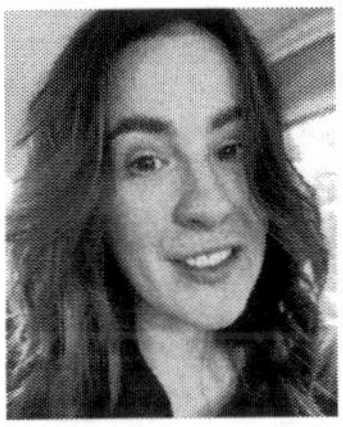

Victoria Shimmens took her undergraduate degree in English Language from Northumbria University in 2012, before travelling and settling in Australia for some time as she worked with grieving families supported by a cancer charity. On returning to the UK, Victoria worked with young autistic women diagnosed with intellectual disabilities and mental health difficulties, before returning to Northumbria University and completing her MSc in Psychology in 2019. She then joined Mental Health Concern, a charity working in partnership with the National Health Service, and then as an assistant psychologist with people with intellectual disabilities and people with severe mental health problems, in the Northeast of England and Yorkshire. Victoria has published articles on the long-term outcomes of people receiving support from community teams, and the language used by these teams. A key reason for publishing this book arose from Victoria's experiences in health and social care which she has seen from several angles – in life experiences, as a voluntary and paid carer, and as a clinician. The importance of trauma-informed care, the need for personal connection over a substantial period of time in order to achieve positive change in people's lives, and overcoming organisational defences, are central to her work.

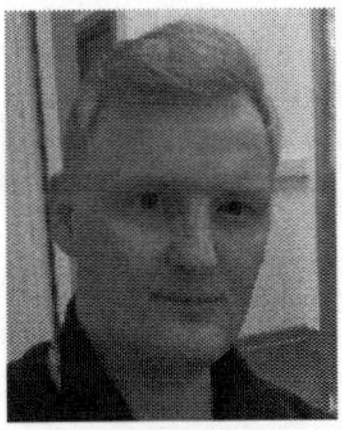

Dr Allan Skelly obtained his first degree in Psychology from the Queen's University of Belfast in 1991, before obtaining a PhD from the University of Warwick in 1996 and a DClinPsych from the University of Surrey in 1998. Allan has worked as a psychologist for people with intellectual disabilities for over 30 years.

Allan was the 2019–2021 Chair of the Faculty for People with Intellectual Disabilities (FPID) of the British Psychological Society (BPS) and is a Consultant Clinical Psychologist practicing in the Northeast of England. Allan has published many articles promoting a focus on the close personal relationships of people with an intellectual disability, the heightened lifetime risk that these will be broken or strained, and how to address this in clinical work. Allan actively promotes the Trauma-Informed Care agenda and the application of attachment theory in doing this. He is the author of published articles and book chapters promoting psychodynamic approaches to people with an intellectual disability (including a controlled trial) as well as applying attachment theory-based interventions in clinical practice. Allan was chair of the working group which produced the 2017 BPS clinical practice guidelines for the integration of attachment theory into the work of clinical psychologists in the UK. As well as reviewing the available clinical tools for formal assessment in several publications, he has collaborated on the design and validation of specific tools for this purpose.

Foreword

Professor Nigel Beail

Reading this book has led me to reflect on my now over 40 year-career working as a clinical psychologist in health services for people who have intellectual disabilities (ID). Firstly, the theories that have informed the work of Allan and Victoria have also informed much of my clinical work and research. Secondly, the accounts of the life experiences of the people in this book seemed familiar to me. It was as if I had met many of them. Of course I have not, but they seem to have a shared experience of many of the people I have worked with. This book therefore helps develop our awareness of the lived experience of people who have ID who access services. Moreover, the book also brings to the fore the issue of love and attachment in the lives of those we support.

My first experiences of working with people who have ID was during my clinical training. I worked under the supervision of an experienced clinical psychologist in a large (what was then called) Mental Handicap Hospital. There were 440 adults and children living in the hospital at that time. As pointed out in this book, a dominant theory in services for people who have ID was behavioural theory. Inspired by a study by Maureen Oswin of children living in long stay hospitals (Oswin, 1978), I decided that I would do my research thesis on one of the children's wards. Taking a behavioural approach, I observed the interactions between the staff and the children when they returned home from school each day. For these children the ward was their home. Behavioural theory would argue that staff should be positively reinforcing the children's positive behaviours to assist their development. Where I used timed observations of staff and child interactions to collect my data, Maureen used participant observation to collect her data. Unfortunately, my study confirmed her findings. We both found the levels of interaction were very low and largely based on meeting the children's physical needs (Beail, 1985; Oswin, 1978). Further to this, Oswin reported only observing five minutes of "mothering" attention (cuddling, play, talking) in a ten-hour period.

At the time I was carrying out these observations, I was also undergoing psychoanalytic supervision with a psychoanalyst with an interest in attachment theory. I found myself being concerned about the children's sense of self and their emotional needs and development. I decided to carry out a further study of children from the same school, but who lived at home. This found the opposite results, in that very high levels of positive interactions were taking place between the child with disabilities and their parents and siblings (Beail, 1988). I concluded that the interactions I observed in family homes were natural, the children were loved and it was unfortunate that such interactions do not occur naturally in hospitals. Fortunately, due to policy changes in the UK all the children moved from the hospital to community-based services by the end of the 1980s. Six children from the hospital moved to a staffed ordinary house in the area I was working in the community, and I carried out an evaluation of this new provision. Levels of interaction between staff and children were found to be much higher but still nowhere near that enjoyed by the children that lived with their parents. I also questioned this new provision by asking how many children live with five other children and are looked after by nurses (Beail, 1989). The staff in the new home all came from the hospital and brought institutional practices with them. The children were not allowed access to all the areas of *their own home*, they did not have their own personal toys or books, and their pictures were not allowed on the walls.

Sadly at that time the ideas of psychoanalytic theorists, which have informed the authors of this book, played little or no role in informing the care and support of people with disabilities. However, my experiences working with people who have ID influenced my career choice and when I qualified, I began work as a clinical psychologist in a community team. I would have happily taken a job at the hospital but none were available, as posts were now being established in the new community teams. I soon found that there was a need to offer psychological interventions to a continuous flow of referrals of people with ID with psychological distress. I began to offer psychodynamically-informed psychotherapy, but found myself apart from my peers who largely worked in the behavioural model. At that time the evidence base for the behavioural approach with people who had ID concerned me, due to its use of punishment to eliminate problem behaviour. However, things were moving, and some were arguing that the behaviours held a communicative function, and that punishment was inappropriate. I decided to explore with my clients what they were trying to communicate through talking therapy. What became apparent quite quickly was that traumatic experiences both experienced in long-stay hospitals and the community were a major theme in clients' discourse.

Concurrently, Valerie Sinason and Pat Frankish were also working this way. They found the same themes and began writing about them (see Beail, 2021). We were also using the theories of Freud, Klein, Bowlby, Mahler and Winnicott, which have been embraced by the authors of this book. In the 1980s our approach and findings were not generally accepted, but as referenced in Chapter 1 the important paper by Mike Bender was published in 1993, which points to the established view of psychoanalytic and other theorists at that time: that people with ID are not suitable for psychotherapy. We had no support from the psychotherapy community, but this eventually led to the formation of the Institute for Psychotherapy and Disability which would provide us with a home and platform. It has taken many years for psychological therapies for people who have ID to become accepted as needed and for the care of those people to become trauma informed.

This raises the central issue. For years people, public bodies, and governments have believed that people who have ID do not need the same things as the rest of the population. Following his research on children living within a London orphanage, John Bowlby promoted the importance of maternal care and the negative impact of maternal deprivation. One negative result of his research and argument was to provide a rationale for women being encouraged to leave the jobs they had held through the Second World War, and to return to being housewives and mothers. Strikingly, his thesis was not applied to those with ID, as many were placed in institutions rather than be supported to live at home, thus breaking their emotional bond and attachment with their parents and loved ones. Living in long stay hospitals did not afford them an ordinary and fulfilling life: their need for love, attention and affection was largely disregarded. Those that remained with their parents were loved but their parents struggled to get the right support. People who have ID were not provided with the same educational opportunities, social care and physical or mental health care as the rest of the population. Adverse Childhood Experiences have also been found to occur at a much higher rate amongst people who have ID, as the authors have shown.

In the 1980s I argued for the development of modes and methods of psychotherapy for people who have ID (Beail, 1984). I was therefore delighted, when I edited the report on psychological therapies for people who have ID three decades later, to see such significant developments in theory and practice (Beail, 2016).

Throughout my career I have been concerned by the interpretation of some of the behaviours of people who have ID as 'attention seeking'. *Love, Attachment and Intellectual Disability* describes how this is still happening, for example in Sonny's case (Chapter 12) the authors give us a different view; he is simply communicating his need for human connection, an attachment, love. This book is therefore a welcome addition to the literature as it has bravely taken the need for love and attachment in the lives of people who have ID as its central theme. The authors promote the view that people who have ID, like everybody else, need love in their life through their attachments to others.

So, as they say, let's put love at the heart of care.

References

Beail, N. (1984). Psychotherapy with mentally handicapped people. *Division of Clinical Psychology Newsletter*. 43, 58-59.

Beail, N. (1985). The nature of interactions between nursing staff and profoundly multiply handicapped children. *Child, Care, Health, and Development*, 11, 113-129

Beail, N. (1988). A comparative observational study of the care provided in hospital with the care provided at home for profoundly multiply handicapped children. *Behavioural Psychotherapy*. 16, 285-296.

Beail, N. (1989). Evaluation of a staffed ordinary house for children with severe learning difficulties. *Child, Care, Health, and Development*. 15, 117-127

Beail, N. (ed.) (2016) Psychological therapies and people who have intellectual disabilities. Leicester: British Psychological Society.

Beail, N. (2021). Freud, psychoanalysis, and trauma: significance in the acknowledgement and identification of trauma in the lives of people who have intellectual disabilities. In N. Beail, P. Frankish & A Skelley. *Trauma and intellectual disability: Acknowledgement, identification, and intervention*. Shoreham by Sea: Pavilion.

Bender, M. (1993). The unoffered chair: The history of therapeutic disdain towards people with a learning difficulty. *Clinical Psychology Forum*. 54, 7-12.

Oswin, M. (1978). *Children living in long-stay hospitals*. London: Heinemann

Preface

One might expect that a book with "Love" in its title would be focused on romantic love in adulthood, the kind that is the focus of many novels, films, documentaries, reality TV shows, and so on. We know that many people with intellectual/learning disabilities place a high value on meeting romantic partners, but as with all their relationships, they are more likely to be maltreated by them and to endure this for longer (McConnell & Phelan, 2022).

This book is not about such romantic love, the problems that society will place in the way of such relationships being attained, or the vulnerabilities and pitfalls of adult courting. This book is about the ***basics*** of love – our earliest attachments that met our basic needs for safety, care, stimulation and adoration. As babies, everyone should experience the kind of love that Freud (1914) called "so moving and at bottom so childish". In this view, parental love is childish, because it forms from the parent's wish to create a person in their own image, only a better version. We should simply drive someone, even if only our mother or father, into an unmitigated joy at our very existence. Of course, we need to move on from this as we develop, to prevent becoming narcissists. Freud's own mother, Amalia Freud, considered him destined for great things, and referred to him as "my golden Sigi". And so he turned out to be, in the sense of his huge impact on the 20th Century. It can reasonably be argued that Freud introduced the idea that talking to a sympathetic person was a better way to treat people suffering from psychological pain, than simply incarcerating them in asylums, leaving them to their family, or abandoning them to destitution.

Bowlby's work, which can be clearly traced back to Freud, picked up on our need for a close, intense, and warm relationship with one or both parents, in order to develop to our potential. Attachment theory suffers from a misnomer, in the sense that it is not 'just a theory'. Bowlby used ethology (the study of animal behaviour) and careful observation of orphans to show that humans can be very badly damaged when they are unloved as infants. This was sadly confirmed by the Romanian orphanage studies after the fall of Ceausescu. Institutionalisation is not good for any child, though for many years people with intellectual disabilities were expected to live in such conditions, which was supported by behavioural psychologists. The behavioural psychologists of the 1950s had little time for Freud or Bowlby, who they considered to be fanciful and unscientific. The modern tradition of behaviourism in Britain, though humane and positive about individual potential, remains sceptical of the importance of attachment, and this can be traced back to its roots in institutional settings.

Much of what we have written in this book may seem very critical of services and the views of individuals and society towards people with intellectual disabilities. Many of our experiences and views are stark and challenging, but we would rather that the truth, as we see it, is put across, because we feel that it is necessary for this to happen.

All the cases and teams presented in this book contain ‘composites’ of at least four people and/or have been heavily disguised for anonymity. Any close similarity to a particular case may be apparent to some readers, but that will be due to the issues presented being so common in clinical practice, or an extreme coincidence. With more than 40 years of experience between us, it was relatively easy for us to access our knowledge of multiple clinical examples to describe each issue presented and to overlay these so that no one should be identifiable.

We hope that readers will grasp our intent to seed a revolution in policy for people with intellectual disabilities. We want family-style care and freedom from childhood maltreatment to be a universal right and championed for these most deserving of people. History will not be kind to the generation who knew that they had to contend with the double whammy of disability in an ableist world on the one hand, and maltreatment on the other, yet who let this situation continue. Emotional security is a right, not a fortunate occurrence for some but not others.

References

Freud S (1914) On Narcissism: An Introduction. In Freud S (1958) The Standard Edition of the Complete Psychological Works of Sigmund Freud, Vol. 14, p.91.

McConnell D, Phelan, S K (2022) Intimate partner violence against women with intellectual disability: A relational framework for inclusive, trauma-informed social services. *Health & Social Care in the Community* **30**, 6, 5156–5166.

Love [luhv]

noun

- a profoundly tender, passionate affection for another person.
- a feeling of warm personal attachment or deep affection, as for a parent, child, or friend.
- sexual passion or desire.

verb (used with object), **loved**, **lov · ing**.

- to have love or affection for
- to have a profoundly tender, passionate affection for (another person).

Attachment [uh-tach-muhnt]

In Psychology:

- an emotional bond between an infant or toddler and primary caregiver, a strong bond being vital for the child's normal behavioural and social development.
- an enduring emotional bond that develops between one person and another in an intimate relationship.

Denial [dih-nahy-uhl]

Noun

- an assertion that something said, believed, alleged, etc., is false.
- refusal to believe a doctrine or theory.
- disbelief in the existence or reality of a thing.
- the refusal to satisfy a claim, request, desire, etc., or the refusal of a person making it.
- refusal to recognize or acknowledge; a disowning or disavowal.

Dictionary.com

Chapter 1: Why this book is needed

"The time is always right to do what is right."

Dr Martin Luther King Jnr., Speech at Oberlin College, 1964

In 1993, Mike Bender wrote a paper for UK clinical psychologists in their professional journal *Clinical Psychology Forum* in which he spoke about 'the unoffered chair'. While it never made the mainstream media, this paper stuck with many of us working in specialist learning disability services. Why were people who had intellectual disabilities not offered the same range of therapies as other people? Training as a counsellor and as a clinical psychologist in the 1990s, Allan Skelly was told by a qualified clinical psychologist that "only simple behavioural conditioning is effective with this group – don't bother with trying to counsel them or their families".

This was a common – *the* common – view among psychologists. 'Behavioural conditioning' refers to the technique of rewarding desired behaviours and punishing undesired behaviours. While punishment-based treatments are now frowned upon as the abuse that they are, there has been little atonement for them by the healthcare services and influential individuals who recommended them as treatment, and the professionals who designed the treatments are still working today. Perhaps this lack of atonement is why electroshock treatments – torture – are still being debated and carried out in the US in 2023.

As a trainee clinical psychologist, Allan Skelly had the benefit of being mentored by Richard Ball, who did not accept this view. Richard could see the value of a counselling model to his team, and supported Allan to do this work on two of five of his days as an assistant psychologist at Gulson Hospital, Coventry. In those days, few believed that psychotherapy, especially psychodynamic psychotherapy, could be effective for people with intellectual disabilities. Speaking to most colleagues about this was either a conversation stopper (and for the practice to be considered somewhat rogue) or would lead to a sudden positive response where the other professional would say that they had often wondered why this situation was allowed. But even with those who responded with positivity

– or even delight – at the idea of counselling for people with intellectual disabilities, few psychologists or psychiatrists in the UK actively supported the use of psychotherapy with people with an intellectual disability.

Several reasons have been put forward for the unoffered chair: that psychotherapy patients needed reasoning ability (as suggested by Freud himself); the general social exclusion of disabled people from public policy and positions of power in society; institutional care not involving any curiosity about personal experience; and the 'medicalisation' of intellectual disability. For many years, children with intellectual disabilities were committed to lifelong care in NHS hospitals, which were chronically underfunded and failed to provide the intimate, reliable and responsive parental care that we would now consider a basic human right. For us, none of these factors really capture the enduring problem of love-deprived lives that many people with intellectual disabilities are forced to endure. Behind the tight paperwork-walls of mental health and learning disability services lurk some very profound, and often dark, feelings about intellectual disability, feelings that do not appear in the letters between professionals, or the minutes of the many meetings we are asked to attend.

We believe that there is a profound wish to avoid looking directly into the lives of people with intellectual disabilities, because what lies there is often extremely painful.

Exceptions prove the rule, however.

In 1983, the first female professor of psychiatry, Joan Bicknell, published 'The Psychotherapy of Mental Handicap' in the *British Journal of Psychiatry*. This has become a seminal paper, calling for family-style care rather than impersonal institutional care for people with intellectual disabilities. Bicknell opposed the forced sterilisation of minors who had an intellectual disability before anyone else; she opposed institutional care as a first resort; she led the committee of enquiry into appalling care at Normansfield Hospital; and she pioneered the multidisciplinary team to manage hospital care as an alternative to the god-like medical superintendents.

Then, in 1992 (updated 2010), Valerie Sinason published 'Mental Handicap and The Human Condition', which exposed the historical denigration of people with intellectual disabilities and how language becomes the vehicle for excluding them from cultural awareness. Several moving case histories illustrated how 'secondary handicap' (either the denial of disability, or an exaggeration of it) could serve to avoid the awareness of the person's pain in living with their disability. The price of being allowed to exist, for many people, is to be asexual, non-aggressive, a fake. But the underlying drives to relate, make sexual and sensual contact, and to compete with others for love and affection remain, and so the person and those around them engage in all sorts of psychological contortions to maintain their blindness. Sinason speaks of unconscious devaluing, even in psychotherapists, noticing how their unconscious contempt could be seen in little differences, like wearing their shabbiest outfit on the day they saw their disabled client. She reminded us that the original meaning of 'stupid' is to be *numbed by grief*. That is, the history of intellectual disability is a history of trauma (Sinason, 2021). Even with loving parents who treasure their child, living with an intellectual disability involves many experiences of failure and daily 'micro-traumas'; being called names, academic failure, being excluded from the attainments that other people make, and often not having a family of their own. Families can also communicate a fundamental disappointment in them, despite loving them. This in turn affects their character, perhaps seeing how their parents have a more unmitigated joy in their siblings, and becoming what Renata, one of the inspirational people who feature in this book, called "being the black sheep of the family".

We have both been influenced by an important paper by Pat Frankish (1989) and her extensive, personally and theoretically informed approach to emotional development in people with intellectual disabilities. Pat Frankish has long advocated for a deeper understanding of the emotional lives of people with learning disability. Pat's contribution has included raising awareness that people with intellectual disabilities are not thought about in terms of their emotional development – in particular, the degree to which they can emotionally separate from their parents and develop a sense of their own separateness – **separation-individuation**. Pat has pointed out that this develops separately from cognitive development, so that some people have a high IQ but struggle to operate separately from their family even as adults. In the 'Frankish model', she considers that this development of individuation involves chronic exposure to trauma as the disability limits each milestone and the person becomes increasingly stuck in their particular stage of separation. To achieve movement forward with this, it is necessary to acknowledge the trauma, empathise, and provide the correct parenting responses that will help the person reach their potential. In doing so, the carer will become aware that much of the imagined 'independence' and 'choice', which is so lauded in learning disability policies and procedures, is just that – imaginary – and they will feel empowered to meet the person at the level at which they are truly needed.

Nigel Beail was one of the first authors that Allan came across, with a clear example of how to work using a psychodynamic model with people who have an intellectual disability in the 1989 publication *Mutual Respect*, which was edited by David Brandon. Professor Beail's work has been the strongest scientific contribution to supporting counselling and psychotherapy for people with intellectual disabilities. With the support of UK colleagues, Professor Beail drew all of the theories and available research together for *Psychological Therapies and People with Intellectual Disabilities* (Beail, 2016), collaborated in outcomes studies showing successful psychotherapy work (e.g. Beail *et al*, 2007) or edited and supported the development of scientific papers. Suffice it to say, the evidence is now strong enough to categorically reject the unoffered chair, in no small way due to this work (see also Chapter 18).

Baroness Sheila Hollins has also been incredibly influential by insisting on a focus on the emotional lives of people with intellectual disabilities, and not just their behaviours and mental disorders. Her role in the *Books Beyond Words* series shows visual depictions of events and features of life that are consistently avoided in conversations with people who have intellectual disabilities, for example, *Am I going to die?*, *Anne has Dementia*, *Getting on with cancer*, *Ron's feeling blue* and *Loving each other safely*. We have made extensive use of these books in our clinical work. As President of the Royal College of Psychiatrists from 2005 to 2008, and later a Life Peer of the House of Lords in the UK, Sheila Hollins has long reminded us that the emotional lives of people with intellectual disabilities must be kept in mind when they are provided with health and social care. Sheila Hollins also has close personal knowledge about the issues that people with disabilities face. Her son, Nigel, has an intellectual disability. The family's struggle to achieve consistent, safe and enjoyable care arrangements for Nigel was shared in an interview for *The Guardian* newspaper. We strongly agree with Professor Hollins that the policy of discharging people from in-patient units to community homes is deeply flawed.

> [this policy] "*...will never work until people understand it's not about a building and a staff team, or rotas and procedures, but about putting somebody like Nigel at the centre of the plans"... I hope Nigel will be so embedded in his community that there will always be people who'll look out for him, love him and care for him after I'm no longer here. That's what every parent wants.*"
>
> Baroness Hollins, speaking in *The Guardian*, 4th June, 2019

Clearly, these inspirational people are motivated by their professionalism, their ethics, and their grasp of science, policy and literature. They understand that people with intellectual disabilities need allies to raise awareness of their situation and the denials and avoidances of their distress and difficulties.

But they are also telling us that love is often – even usually – compromised in the lives of people with intellectual disabilities.

In 2004, Professor Hollins was involved in a UK-wide survey of psychotherapies in learning disability services by the Royal College of Psychiatrists. In fact, a surprising number of psychiatrists, psychotherapists and psychologists reported that they were engaged in psychotherapy, despite this not being a priority for the National Health Service and its national leadership teams. There were 448 responses to the survey, which is encouraging, as the actual workforce providing therapy is likely to be larger than this sample. Most of these involved reports of positive experiences of offering psychotherapy in one form or another (cognitive behavioural, psychodynamic, family therapy, cognitive analytic, other).

Access to psychological therapies has only burgeoned since that time (Beail, 2016). It seems that, despite the unoffered chair, many people working in health services offer it anyway – and it seems they will not be dissuaded from making the offer. We think this is because they have realised that it is an unforgivable omission – an unconscionable discrimination.

It is time for access to psychotherapy to become a right for people with intellectual disabilities, for it to be expected from their community and hospital services, and for it to end as a fringe activity. In addition, the valuable principles and features of psychotherapeutic thought have to become part of the basic ethos of health and social care. It is not enough to be washing, cleaning, working, going to the leisure centre and watching TV. Someone should love you, delight in you and consider you important in their life; there should be a deep and enduring connection to people you can rely on to be there when times are difficult, and share the joys of life with you.

Who should read this book?

While this book describes work done under the banner of community health services and specifically, a psychology team, it is relevant to all health and social care professionals who help people with intellectual disabilities. We hope it will also be of value to advocates, service commissioners, families and healthcare generalists. Much of what we believe about the importance of attachment theory is relevant to people without intellectual disabilities and could be applied to any group which struggles to find a strong voice in the public sphere.

While we have asked experts by experience to review the themes of this book informally, we are aware that the language used is not very accessible to most people with intellectual disabilities. We recognise that we have additional work to do, beyond writing this book, to share our work directly with the people we want to help. It can be a difficult balance between getting a message across and fully explaining ideas that are inherently complex. Our Emotional Development Workbook[1] is written to be accessible to carers, and we also have a range of accessible materials in our clinical work that we have based on the ideas presented.

We all need someone to love us, deeply. Health and Social Care policy and practice urgently need to address why many, if not most, people with intellectual disabilities are not loved and valued in the same uncomplicated way that others are. Simply referring people to short psychological therapies and teaching 'coping techniques', such as breathing or mindfulness techniques, behavioural interventions, or medication, are not enough, and can often be harmful. While these options can be helpful for some people, we have noted that many of the people we see who feel profoundly unloved, or even unworthy of love, have had them before. Their memory of these interventions is not of what technique they were taught or their precise medication dosage, but their experience

1 For more information, please contact the authors via the publisher. Appropriate use by professionals, families and carers will be considered open access.

of the person who spoke with them – whether they were welcoming and warm, or cold, rejecting, quick to 'discharge' them; whether they were understanding and empathic, or concerned with their own agenda and the need for the person to 'get better' or 'behave well'.

> *"I've learned that people will forget what you said, people will forget what you did, but people will never forget how you made them feel."*
>
> Attributed to Maya Angelou

References

Beail N (ed) (2016) *Psychological Therapies and People with Intellectual Disabilities*. Report of the Royal College of Psychiatrists and the British Psychological Society. London: Royal College of Psychiatrists.

Bicknell J (1983) The psychopathology of handicap. *British Journal of Medical Psychology*, **56**, 167-178.

Bender M (1993) The unoffered chair: the history of therapeutic disdain towards people with a learning difficulty. *Clinical Psychology Forum* **7** (1) 54.

Beail N (1989) Understanding Emotions: the Kleinian approach explained. In Brandon, D. (ed). *Mutual respect: Therapeutic approaches to working with people with learning difficulties*. Surrey: Good Impressions.

Frankish P (1989) Meeting the emotional needs of handicapped people: a psychodynamic approach. *Journal of Mental Deficiency Research* **33** 407-14.

Royal College of Psychiatrists (2004) *Psychotherapy and Learning Disability*. Council CR116 Report. London: Royal College of Psychiatrists.

Sinason V (2021) The history of disability is a history of trauma. In Frankish, P., Beail, N. & Skelly, A. (eds) *Trauma and Intellectual Disability: Acknowledgement, Identification and Intervention*. West Sussex: Pavilion Publishing.

Sinason V (1992/2010) *Mental Handicap and the Human Condition: An Analytic Approach to Intellectual Disability*. London: Free Association Books.

Chapter 2: Theories of our need for love

Klein, Mahler, Bowlby and Došen

"We must begin to love in order not to fall ill."

Sigmund Freud, *On Narcissism*, 1925

In one sense, our modern understanding of the need for love goes back to Freud. Freud's original theories of neurosis and personality were focused on how the internal 'drives' (for sex and competitive aggression) are acted out in families when we are children. While he was very interested in the conduct of the parents as remembered by his patients, the essential difficulty was overcoming the love *complexes* that arose within the minds of the patients that he tried to help.

Freud was focused, not without criticism, on the possessive, early 'sensual-sexual' feelings that we have at various stages of development. We are 'oral' when we are focused on our need for our mother's breast; we are 'anal' when we are trying to get control of our bowels; we are 'phallic' when we notice our genitalia and start to explore them; and we are 'genital' when we start to guess about how this genitalia could interact with others. However, as children, we receive the message that these comments about 'willies' and 'boobies' are not allowed – you should not talk about them. You should not try to work out if you will be a mummy or a daddy yourself, or what mummies and daddies do when they are in the bedroom alone. Consciously, this is about learning where you are in the family. For a time, between about five and eleven years, you are in a curiously non-sexual stage, called 'latency'. You are compliant, find people kissing 'yeuch', and are working on being a 'good boy' or 'good girl'. Then we hit adolescence and the hormonal revolution that re-activates all of our previous memories and thoughts from childhood, which we start to apply in our own rehearsals for romantic relationships.

Freud contended that traumatic experiences, such as parental divorce or death, would strongly affect the personality according to what age the person is when such events take place. He proposed the idea of emotional trauma to determine where such events would be expected to 'arrest' development or lead to an unhelpful focus later in life. He noticed that many of his patients reported sexual abuse by their parents, and the earlier this began, the more damaging it appeared to be. He has been criticised for forsaking this theory (Masson, 1984) in favour of the idea that the abuse was fantasised, but later returned to trauma as a cause of neurosis.

In *Beyond the Pleasure Principle* (1920), Freud defined trauma as perceiving an event or events as breaking through a 'protective shield' which normally keeps out the things we need not think about so that we can get on with loving and working. When an event is too horrible, the shield is broken down, so that all we can do is experience the traumatic event over and over, finding ourselves bound to the event with no way to consign it to the past. In some of his cases, such events were literally unthinkable. Hence their *conversion* into the strange physical ailments that he described. Even today, the British Medical Association estimated that 20% of new consultations to general practitioners, 52% of new referrals to secondary care, and 20-25% of frequent attenders at medical clinics have medically unexplained symptoms (Jadhakan *et al*, 2019).

We now know that sexual abuse is a common cause of later and often complex psychological difficulties, though even Freud found this hard to believe. While traumatic events in adulthood can be enough to create a post-traumatic reaction needing help, early trauma, neglect and adversity are hugely important risk factors for the severity and course of psychological distress.

Melanie Klein

Melanie Klein (nee Reizes; 1882-1960) built on the theories of Freud, but unlike Freud, she believed that children could and should be offered clinical help with their emotions. Born in Vienna, she had wanted to be a doctor, but this was not possible for married women at the time – Melanie had married Arthur Klein at the age of 21. Melanie was unhappy with married life and was very excited by Freud's ideas, which stimulated her interest and helped her overcome feelings of depression. She presented a study of her son Erich to the Hungarian Psychoanalytic Society in 1919 and was offered membership. Later, she attended psychoanalytic conferences and practised in Berlin, but the connections she made in London became lasting and she had a huge effect on British psychotherapy as a field of study and practice.

In 1923, she offered daily sessions to a young girl, which resulted in a paper, *The Development of a Child*. Developing child analysis in Berlin, her marriage finally ended in 1924. The famous 'Bloomsbury Group' from London befriended her, seeking radical new and modern ideas. After moving to London in 1926 at the invitation of the analyst Earnest Jones, she began to analyse a small group of patients including her friends and their family. She did not shy away from very unhappy children, including children diagnosed with schizophrenia like 'Dick', although nowadays this would be described as a form of autism. This work led to ideas about 'symbol formation', which refers to the need for children to be able to play and pretend in order to be happy, but they need to have an emotional connection in order to give this play some meaning (many children on the spectrum of autism can engage in pretend play, but do not choose to do so because they are unable to rehearse social interactions within this play). What Klein did with Dick, over a very long period of time, was to remain attentive and present despite his great difficulty in connecting with her and understanding his emotional world.

One of Klein's major books, *The Psycho-Analysis of Children* (1932), demonstrated that analysing children could be done and could really help children manage the terrible anxieties that they can feel. It also demonstrated that children have hugely dramatic emotional states and need steady responses from adults that involve no retribution or withdrawal. By doing so, and adopting the therapist's 'stance', children eventually learn that the dramas, fears and setbacks they experience are survivable, do not lead to catastrophe, and that people will not try to annihilate them because they have lashed out, when scared or envious. Such experiences of the present, non-retributive, and 'non-sulky' adult are necessary for a person to experience tolerable anxiety in their life.

We could not agree with Klein more on this point. What if this need is lifelong? We believe that this is an important part of love; the patient, continuing, listening, and empathic presence of someone emotionally wiser, stronger in emotional terms, and kind.

Klein's theory includes the concepts of the ***paranoid-schizoid*** and ***depressive*** positions. They are 'positions' because it is very easy to regress from the latter to the former. Depressive refers not to unrealistic depression (because depressed people are usually far harder on themselves than is realistic) but the sense of loss and deflation, but also relief in realising that the world is not as terrible as we thought – that the people who love us can also be irritable, spiteful or unfair – and to experience the 'whole' of them at the same time, rather than denigrating one moment and hating them the next.

The paranoid-schizoid position is also necessary, but not the state of mind we would wish to stay in. It is formed because we need to be able to 'split' our experience when we first feed – in order to feed trustingly, a baby can move immediately from a state of hungry agony to a blissful experience of receiving milk. However, babies cannot determine where the mother's glands or their bottle end and the person begins. What they feel about their feeding, they also feel about the other. And this is the basis of our understanding of others. We start, over time, to notice that the parent who frustrates, withholds, shouts at us, or does not make us comfortable quickly enough when we have discharged our bodily fluids, is also the person who satisfies, cares, comforts and delights in us. This allows us to start to remember this, and as we grow, we lose the 'ideal' experience but gain a more realistic sense of the other. This is disappointing but hopeful.

Children whose care is less than good can struggle to stop the paranoid-schizoid position from dominating the development of their personality. Where there is outright abuse, they may become very disoriented and even seem to find it difficult to contact reality. Child maltreatment is now very clearly linked to many forms of poor health outcomes, something which the psychoanalysts knew well from the beginning of the 20th Century. Yet, this obvious but hidden need for warmth and love in childhood did not become culturally accepted until the writings of John Bowlby around the time of the Second World War, who himself was analysed by Melanie Klein.

Margaret Mahler

Margaret Mahler (nee Schönberger; 1897-1985) was a Jewish Hungarian psychoanalyst who was educated in Budapest and Munich, but eventually went to Vienna to be trained by Helene Deutsch after meeting the Hungarian psychoanalyst Sándor Ferenczi. She worked as an analyst until she married Paul Mahler in 1936 and moved to the United States in 1938.

Unlike Klein, Mahler believed in working with children and parents together. At the Masters Children's Centre in Manhattan, Mahler attempted to help very unhappy children and noticed that they were often very badly treated by others. She documented the effects on children of early separation from their mothers and noticed that this coincided with poor development of a realistic idea of other people (object-representations) and even more disturbed ideas of themselves (self-representations).

In *The Psychological Birth of the Human Infant* (1975), Mahler proposed that we develop a sense of separateness in the early years of life, beginning with a sense of being joined to our parent. There are distinct phases of this separation process, as follows:

1. **Symbiosis:** the child is aware of the parents, but there is no sense of being an individual. The child's frustration is partly because the parents will not meet their needs immediately. However, the child does have an awareness that there is an 'out there' that is not the parents.
2. **Hatching:** The child starts to see the parents as separate, with increased awareness and interest in the outside world. The parents are the 'point of orientation' and the child engages in a lot of eye contact.
3. **Practising:** at about nine to 16 months, the child can crawl about and then walk. They start to explore actively and assume the presence of the parents without realising their own separateness. Because of this, there can be rages when the world does not fit the child's expectations.
4. **Rapprochement:** typically, at about 15 months, the child starts to realise that, when they wander away from their parent, there is separateness. Initially, there is an exploration of what objects will do, such as pushing them over or dropping them. As rapprochement progresses with language and the ability to refer to remote objects, the ability to share attention to additional people and objects (triads) becomes available. It is very important in this stage to support the child in their explorations, as if the parent is unavailable or intermittent, the world will become an anxious place because support cannot be relied upon.

Mahler also talked about the concept of object constancy, meaning that the child understands that parents are separate individuals with their own intentions and wishes. If the relationship with others is not positive, the child learns that others are a source of anxiety, not a source of support and solace. This becomes a powerful basis of the person's personality and experience of mental well-being, or, alternatively, excessive distress or anxiety.

Disability Psychotherapy was founded by Dr Pat Frankish, focusing on the Mahler stages in people whose development is significantly limited by learning disability. The assessment essentially involves identifying where a person may be partially or wholly arrested in an earlier phase of separation-individuation. Entirely separate from the person's cognitive (intellectual) development, the person's emotional development can be determined by how their behaviour in an observation best matches a particular stage of separation-individuation. Frankish and colleagues contend that the person can be supported, through a therapeutic relationship, to move towards the next stage. As well as this, expectations can be adjusted to be more appropriate, usually to an earlier stage than carer expectations suggest, as people with intellectual disabilities.

The Frankish Assessment is available to buy for professionals with prior expertise in healthcare for people with intellectual disabilities from Pavilion Publishing or Frankish Training Ltd (www.frankishtraining.co.uk).

John Bowlby

John Bowlby (1907 - 1990) was born into an upper-class family. His father was a famous and successful doctor, with a knighthood and royal connections. As a young child, Bowlby was cared for by a nanny, Minnie, until the age of four. He would see his mother, Mary, for only one hour after teatime, as, among upper-class families of this time, it was believed that too much parental attention and affection would lead to a dangerous spoiling of children.

Also in line with class expectations, Minnie's care was ended when he was four years old, and replaced by a shared nanny who was remembered as cruel and sarcastic. At the age of seven, Bowlby was sent to boarding school where parental warmth was explicitly discouraged in favour of gender segregation and a rigorous and punitive regime, encouraging obedience to school masters and older boys. Surprisingly to the modern reader, Bowlby actually supported the idea of boarding school for much of his career, but then changed his mind decisively. In 1973, he declared that "I wouldn't send a dog away to boarding school age seven". When he wrote this, it was normal for people with intellectual disabilities to live in segregated special hospitals, where their behaviour was modified by powerful medications and behaviour-modification techniques, including punishments that would now be considered cruel and degrading. Psychologists working in these 'Mental Handicap Hospitals' were uncomfortable with Bowlby's ideas about the necessity of family-style care, though, eventually, heroic innovators like Dr Joan Bicknell called for it (Bicknell, 1983), and while such voices are often ignored, they have never and will never be silenced. Nowadays, large institutions are no more, but smaller care arrangements continue to have the potential to become cruel and degrading – one of the main reasons we have written this book.

Bowlby studied medicine at Cambridge, but left because his main interest was developmental psychology, taking up a job in a school. He then studied psychology and pre-clinical science at Trinity College, graduating at the age of 26. He then studied psychiatry at the Maudsley Hospital, and in 1936 qualified as a psychoanalyst. His careful work with deprived orphans in the Canonbury Clinic during the war taught him that early deprivation of maternal care was associated with a lack of affection for others and petty criminality. As a result of this and other studies, Bowlby published *Maternal Care and Mental Health* (1951), which was published by the World Health Organisation.

> *"...the infant and young child should experience a warm, intimate and continuous relationship with his mother (or mother substitute)."*
>
> John Bowlby, 1951

This, and an influential film with James Roberston entitled *A Two Year Old Goes to Hospital* (1952), led to significant changes in the practices involved in children's healthcare, ending the practice of excluding the parents from children's wards. Unhappy with previous theories, Bowlby went on to develop attachment theory, the theory that interruptions in or coldness and cruelty in caring for children were a main basis of human suffering.

Mary Ainsworth and colleagues later developed the *Strange Situation* technique to determine, at age one year, what their attachment pattern will be. There will be one of three types of 'Attachment Strategy':

- Children will become relatively secure if they are constitutionally well, are attended to, and are interacted with by understanding, empathic parents, and are comforted and reassured when they hurt themselves or become worried. They are more likely to become confident, optimistic and sociable adults.

- Children will become over-anxious if their parents are intermittently available to them or their moods are hard to predict. They will become preoccupied adults with problems in self-esteem and relationships, and will expect that others will not be there for them. They value relationships, but their personal story is painful and involving.
- Children will become relatively aloof and not wish to discuss their feelings if their parent is too strict, rejecting or punitive when they express themselves. They will become avoidant adults who act out distress, have physical symptoms of stress, or who deny that talking about feelings has any value. They will avoid showing their feelings and struggle to express themselves in relationships, sometimes becoming hostile or 'dismissing' when others need them to be attentive.

Later, a fourth type of response to incomplete or abusive parenting was added, known as Disorganisation of attachment. Where parents are outright frightening, or where childhood is marked by several adversities, the person will become convinced that the very people we need care from are not to be trusted and relationships will be avoided. The person is more likely to have low self-esteem, marked mental health problems, and perhaps even the feeling that they are unworthy of love itself.

Anton Došen

Anton Došen (1939 - 2023) was an emeritus professor of the psychiatry of intellectual disability at Radboud University, Nijmegen, Netherlands. With over 40 years' experience in the field, Professor Došen was for a decade the Chair of the Intellectual Disability section of the World Health Organisation and founded the European Association for Mental Health in Intellectual Disability (EAMHID), and was honorary President of the Association. Professor Došen's work emphasises the need for an understanding of emotional development (independent of cognitive development and the development of living skills).

Emotional development as proposed by Došen is well described in Sappok *et al*'s (2021) *Meeting Emotional Needs in Intellectual Disability.* Došen proposes that development follows a series of necessary stages:

1. **Adaptation** (Symbiosis), in the first six months of life there is a physical and emotional 'unity' between the individual and their caregiver, with the world perceived primarily through the senses of smell, taste, touch, hearing and temperature. The aim is homeostasis – not feeling too cold, or hot, not being hungry or thirsty, and not over- or under-stimulated. The person has no ability to communicate different forms of discomfort, so crying serves to communicate all of these. Carers should be close, organise events and stimulation, and be vigilant for discomfort or distress, the source of which they may need to guess. They must be what Sappok and colleagues call the *Reliable Provider*. Self-injury, for example, is an appeal, an expression of need. There is no object permanence or constancy. That is to say, when a person is out of sight, they seem to have really disappeared, which can be very frightening. The person is very vulnerable to the emotional state of the carer, and emotional contagion is very likely. For example, a care team who feels depressed and hopeless in the face of distressing self-injury may lead the person to also feel helpless and joyless. In adults with an intellectual disability functioning at this level, the world continues to be experienced through the body and immediate surroundings, and it is therefore developmentally normal to self-stimulate by rocking, flapping hands or masturbating.
2. **Socialisation** (Safety), from about seven to 18 months, where the person is still very dependent on their carer to explore the world, but an attachment bond is formed that allows the person to explore more widely. Anger, joy, sadness and fear become recognisably different from each other to adult carers. The world is explored through touch, such as by pushing objects, manipulating them and moving towards and away from them (and people) with increasing competence. The person gains object permanence (or object *constancy*; the confidence that people and things which move out of view still exist). A person starts to understand that they have a separate body from other people, but is still confused about separateness, and is egocentric. There is a strong focus on main carers and little interest in peers. Siblings or peers who seem to distract the main carers are targets for aggression. The person is fearful of separation and loss of caregivers, but cannot rein

in their frustration; this can cause tension on the bond with the carer. Parental or carer anger in response to repeated physical aggression from the child can be a source of carer guilt, but constancy in the carers' commitment tends to win out, strengthening the bond over the longer term. For adults with intellectual disabilities who remain at this stage of development, aggression and self-harm risk being seen as sentient, conscious and deliberate, especially as it seems to meet the person's wishes (e.g. to gain or retain interaction, to avoid demands) at the 'expense' of the carer's safety or feelings.

3. **First individuation** (Autonomy-seeking) leading to a sense of separateness or basic autonomy, from about 19 months to three years of age. Being able to explore more widely, the child is now easily excited, but also rather easily frustrated. It is less important that a topic is discussed or an activity completed than the person has a sense that they can influence the topic or activity, and that their separate will is recognised. This phase can be very challenging, because the person both wishes to break free of the caregiver to an extent, but also relies heavily on them. They have an emotional language, and can refer to their internal state, though this is incomplete and still requires some interpretation by the carer. As yet, they are unable to see that people who criticise them or frustrate them still love them. The person discovers that they have an independent will and don't have to follow what the carer wants, but lack empathy with others. When placed with peers, they will play alongside them rather than interact with them. The person will not know the difference between conviction and facts – the person is not 'deluded', rather they don't yet realise that what is true is different from what is imagined. Moral reasoning and the resulting self-restraint cannot yet be expected from the person, and new skills are not learned when strains are very stressful, e.g. being rebuked when screaming with frustration cannot teach the person to avoid screaming, just as a drowning person is not learning to swim. For adults with intellectual disabilities functioning at this level, providing care can be difficult when the person wants something to happen but cannot accept that this is not possible. They can respond with aggression when thwarted, and while distressed at the hurt caused to carers, struggle to integrate this into proper empathy. Their partial understanding of their behaviour and emotions may make aggression seem premeditated, placing strain upon the bond with carers, who may be at risk of actual injury. Behavioural conditioning programmes, while helpful for many,

can be hard to maintain and may be unrealistic, given that some aggression is to be expected at this developmental level. It should be remembered that the person's main fear at this level is that they will be denied their sense of agency (self-determination) and just have to do what others tell them.

4. **Identification** (forming the self), which corresponds to the start of formal schooling (four to seven years). The emotional connection to the caregiver should be strong when development has gone well. There is some interest in other children now, and the person can function in groups. The person starts to describe what sort of person they are, e.g. by trying on clothes with pretend connotations, playing a sport, or otherwise placing oneself in a certain grouping. Male or female roles are tried out, e.g. by dressing as a particular hero, or putting on parents' make-up or clothes. Intense fantasy stories can be very common in younger children, and, over time, the difference between what is real and what is imagined (or pretence) becomes apparent. Important steps in 'mentalisation' (being able to imagine someone else's mental perspective and needs) occur in this stage, which, if attained, can greatly enhance the person's future prospects of living in relative autonomy. Children in this phase gain confidence from producing models or other creations, often presenting the adults in the family with gifts they have made. They are very responsive to praise for successful formal learning, but can also risk distress if they feel their creation is not sufficiently beautiful or valuable. It is only at this stage that abstract social rules can be accepted and overrule the person's heartfelt desire, independent of sanction or reward. Alternatives to the preferred activity or object can be accepted at this stage, as the person can now process disappointment, and has the idea of 'no one's fault'. Adults with intellectual disabilities who achieve this stage are less likely to have longstanding histories of challenging behaviours, and when such behaviour occurs it is likely to be related to a personal crisis (such as bereavement or other traumatic event), involving *regression* (going backwards temporarily). Peer contact is sought at this stage and enjoyed. However, adults with intellectual disabilities may seek contact with peers of the same developmental age, which is then misconstrued as sexually inappropriate behaviour, and carers may have to limit such contact, which can be a loss for the individual concerned.

5. **Reality awareness** (Self-differentiating), which occurs from about age eight to age 12. In this stage, we find that logical, rational thinking predominates. The person begins to be able to self-regulate any distress and to have clearly stated moral rules. They can compromise and understand the limits to carers' ability to meet their needs. The person develops a realistic assessment of their strengths and abilities, but may find competition highlights weaknesses that they do not like and which affect their self-esteem. The conscience is well developed and the person lives without regular moral guidance from carers. The person needs some recognition for their status and can actively seek peer relationships that may become lifelong friendships, which the person can maintain, being able to think and respond to the feelings and needs of others. Adults with intellectual disabilities may actually function in independent living arrangements, but may struggle with future planning, and may want the company of carers for reassurance and to check in at times of stress or trauma (e.g. when bereaved, or if they experience discrimination in the community). Carers should remember that most eight-12 year olds are not asked to live in their own flat and deal with all of the vagaries of adult life. They should not mistake object permanence, the ability to function in peer groups, and a wish for autonomy, as an equivalent to the functioning of adults without intellectual disabilities.
6. **Social individuation** (Forming identity) which is seen from about 13 years to adulthood. This phase was added by Sappok *et al* (2021) as Došen's model ends at stage 5, which would correspond to an appropriate level of emotional development to be obtained by a person with a mild intellectual disability (prior to the 12-year level). In this stage, it is proposed that the person will truly seek their own identity and independence. They will be able to find a role in society, usually achieve employment, and find their personal identity They will have friendships, acquaintances and close relationships, with a full range of interests, including entirely new experience-seeking, such as going to a new country. They will, however, still fear being seen as incompetent, worthless or useless, and being excluded from society.

Sappok *et al* (2021) showed how a structured and standardised test[2], the Scale of Emotional Development (SED), can be applied to ascertain the stage of emotional development as originally proposed by Anton Došen.

2 A *standardised* test is one that is shown to be scientifically reliable, and to measure what it says that it measures (scientifically valid).

By accurately identifying the person's level of functioning emotionally, it is then possible for signs of distress or disturbance (e.g. in descriptions of 'challenging behaviour') to be placed in their developmental context. It can then be judged if the expectation that such behaviours should be corrected or extinguished (e.g. by conditioning responses from others) is realistic, or even desirable.

Why we need a new framework to understand people with intellectual disabilities

Theories of the need for love are essential in understanding the lives of people with intellectual disabilities. This book shows many instances of requests for psychological help that occur when carers cannot cope with the impact of chronic emotional or behavioural distress, and the bond with the person becomes threatened or compromised. We contend that, without the perspectives of Freud, Mahler, Frankish, Bowlby and Došen, this strain can and does lead to potentially unhelpful explanations of such signs. We are very concerned about two widely used frameworks for interpreting signs of limited emotional development because of the assumptions they make about the main causes of distress in human beings, and their practice which tries to eliminate certain actions on the grounds of social unacceptability, a slippery and culturally relative process at the best of times.

Psychiatric classification systems

Firstly, we are concerned that insecure attachment and trauma responses are often interpreted within psychiatric classification systems that (i) assign a stigmatising and unreliable label, such as 'bipolar disorder', 'hallucinations' or 'anxiety disorder', and (ii) lead naturally and without challenge to the use of psychotropic medications, which are often designed for people with extreme psychotic experiences (e.g. risperidone, quetiapine, olanzapine), or people who are depressed (e.g. fluoxetine, amytriptyline, venlafaxine). In each of these cases, the realisation that the person's behaviours and emotions can be normal for their stage of emotional development or attachment patterns, and often, in response to exposure to Adverse Childhood Experiences (ACEs), should lead us to be alarmed at the use of such drugs, given their known side effects, which can be irreversible. Not only will the person become known as having an 'illness' that requires lifelong treatment by medication, but there will be an expectation of a 'cure', which will then be endlessly sought. In our experience, the cure is elusive, and a lifetime of dependency on drugs ensues, with great difficulty in phasing the medication out, even when clearly ineffective.

Positive Behaviour Support

Secondly, we are concerned that the Positive Behaviour Support (PBS) movement, admittedly a great advance on the psychiatric classification model, lacks trauma-awareness, attachment-awareness, and developmental perspective. PBS is based on a mixture of ethical principles of equality as espoused in Social Role Valorisation or SRV (including the assumption that, with the right environment, the person will not demonstrate challenging behaviour), added to the technology of Applied Behaviour Analysis, which is basically the shaping of behaviour by the application of reward or punishment in response to a 'target' behaviour. While punitive methods are a thing of the past in the UK (though still well within living memory; see Skelly, 2019), PBS offers false hope for the eventual extinction or redundancy of challenging behaviours through a mixture of avoiding 'triggers' and rewarding 'functionally equivalent behaviours' while ignoring the challenging behaviours. This is extremely hard to achieve in real-world settings, and in the long term is rather ineffective; hence, even PBS advocates consider it a 'model for life'. Short training programmes in PBS do not lead to its competent use (Strydom *et al*, 2020). There is much spontaneous improvement without PBS; lack of awareness prevents access to PBS programmes; and many people who receive PBS are re-referred for the same behavioural issues months or years after their initial referral.

PBS does have some positive features– it does not imply that chemical or brain dysfunction is necessary for behavioural difficulties to arise, there are indeed many environmental adjustments that can address specific behavioural issues, and PBS is also extremely mindful of personal equality and the need for clear, evidence-based assessment. We do feel, however, that PBS risks becoming a movement that ignores evidence that shows its limitations. It can be very difficult to find any studies about the relapse that clinicians see all the time when trying to use PBS. Not only this, but it is often implemented in specialist community teams where the medical model is applied at the same time, which can lead to opposing ideas, confusion and considerable bad feeling between professionals. Some roles have been traditionally associated with medication-based approaches (such as community nursing and psychiatry) while others have been associated with behaviourism (e.g. clinical psychology, Applied Behaviour Analysis) leading to 'turf wars'.

Neither the medical model nor PBS have much, if anything, to say about:

- our developmental needs
- the caregiving acts of our parents that promote or prevent the development of emotional security
- how intellectual disability and its concomitant traumas and adversities complicate the parent-child relationship
- how behaviours inappropriate for a person's chronological age can be appropriate for their level of emotional development.

That is to say, at this time, they have little or nothing to say about our need to be loved in our early life.

What follows is a series of chapters that focus on the life of a particular individual. We present individual sessions as they occurred in some cases, while for others we describe our take on the development of our work across many sessions. Most of this work is individually focused, but some is focused on carers, healthcare systems and organisations. We always think about how the wider system is treating the person, responding as systems of care do, to the conscious but also unconscious wishes of the person themselves, the people around them, the healthcare system intended to support them, and society itself. Readers will note – possibly with some distress – how raw and urgent we have found this work, but will also see that, despite the widespread ignorance and even denial of the effects of love on well-being, and where love is painfully lacking, it is possible to do something about this.

References

Bicknell J (1983) The psychopathology of handicap. *British Journal of Medical Psychology*, **56** 167-178.

Bowlby J (1951) *Maternal Care and Mental Health*. Geneva, Switzerland: World Health Organisation.

Bowlby J (1973) Separation: *Anxiety & Anger. Attachment and Loss* (vol. 2); (International psycho-analytical library no.95). London: Hogarth Press.

Frankish P (2019) *Frankish Assessment of the Impact of Trauma in Intellectual Disabilty (FAIT).* West Sussex: Pavilion Publishing.

Freud S (1920) *Beyond the Pleasure Principle*. London: Karnac Books.

Jadhakhan F, Lindner O, Blakemore A & Gurthrie E (2019) Prevalence of medically unexplained symptoms in adults who are high users of health care services: a systematic review and meta-analysis protocol. *British Medical Journal* Open: https://doi:10.1136/bmjopen-2018-02792

Klein M (1932) *The Psycho-Analysis of Children*. London: Hogarth Press.

Mahler S, Pine F & Bergman A (1973) *The Psychological Birth of the Human Infant*. New York: Basic Books.

Masson J (1984) *The Assault on Truth: Freud's Suppression of the Seduction Theory*. New York: Farrer, Straus & Giroux.

Sappok T, Zepperitz S & Hudson M (2021) *Meeting Emotional Needs in Intellectual Disability.* Hogrefe Publishers.

Skelly A (2019) Historical Myopia and Behaviourism in Clinical Psychology. *Clinical Psychology Forum* **316** 32-35.

Strydom A, Bosco A, Vickerstaff V *et al* (2020) Clinical and cost effectiveness of staff training in the delivery of Positive Behaviour Support (PBS) for adults with intellectual disabilities, autism spectrum disorder and challenging behaviour - randomised trial. *BioMedCentral Open*, **20**, 161.

Chapter 3: Lesley

The failure of attunement

"Being surrounded by the wrong people is the loneliest thing in the world."

Kim Culbertson

This chapter is a description of a home visit by Victoria Shimmens. It describes how failing to attend to the emotional states of a person can lead them to feel alone and helpless, even when surrounded by people. Lesley is a woman in her 20s with a significant learning disability. She communicates mainly with single words, outstretched arms, and occasionally by hurting others, especially when she feels lonely, or ignored.

I had never been to the home before. Mainly, this was because of COVID, but a feeling has always been communicated to us that our visit is unnecessary. Even when I went there, I didn't feel particularly welcome. The person who opened the door was polite, but I was quickly passed to another person from Lesley's team (Alessa). She had met me three times but introduced herself as though we had never met. I was ushered to where Lesley was, in a lounge behind a closed door.

Lesley was sat in the room by herself with headphones on. The door to the room had been shut. She had just been left in the room by herself; she was left to 'self-occupy'. She was prompted to say hello to me, which is not an expectation I have, but she was told to do it. I introduced myself directly to Lesley with a "hello", but it was like that throughout – "Tell Victoria 'hello'". Instructions or mandatory questions: "Are you going to [say hello, tell Victoria about this and that]. It was as though I had to be part of this three-way lie, that everything was okay. Early in our conversation, Alessa said, "What were you hoping to achieve today?" I responded, while being acutely aware of Lesley listening too, that I wanted to come and see how things were going and that I didn't have a fixed agenda. The staff member then kept revisiting this idea of 'achieving something', asking me if I wanted to go through the documentation as though there *had* to be an agenda for the visit, but I resisted this and consistently responded that she should not worry about that and should just "go about their normal day".

But it wasn't like that. There had to be an interview because there was no activity to observe. If I was observing a normal day, staff would not be there, and Lesley would be left to stimulate herself.

So the interview began. I was sat on the same sofa as Lesley, my body language facing both of them. In this triangle, they seemed to compete for the connection with me. They kept talking over each other. Alessa tried to comment on the things Lesley was saying to give me the "correct version of events", as she called it. I felt like she didn't want Lesley to freely let her mind wander to the experiences that she was processing. She was directed back to specific things that the staff were focused on that were a problem for *them*.

They said, "We found that the best routine is to go for walks" and therefore the whole of her daily activity was to go for a walk. This could be for up to a few hours. This would happen when the staff wanted, not when Lesley requested it; in fact, she seemed to have lost the ability to initiate meaningful activities that engaged with her environment. They said, "That's when we see the most behaviours… when we return from the walk", so I commented that this was when there isn't as much to do formally. Alessa then commented about the behavioural intervention requiring an update, as it "had not worked".

In response to this, I began to talk about additional advice that was forthcoming from the community team about her daily structure of activity. However, I also said that there were important things to discuss that were not covered by her behaviour plan, such as emotional needs.

I didn't carry on with this tack, because Lesley kept wanting to talk about her past, her school and people she has known. She was almost reliving it. She said there was a place she loved, but she had to leave "because of money". She talked about a girl she went to school with. Alessa said, "She used to pull your hair, didn't she?" and Lesley said, "Yes, she pulled my hair". By way of demonstrating this, she held her head and whimpered. But then Alessa spoke of a person Lesley ended up living with, who later died. What followed was Alessa spelling out the word 'D-I-E-D' to prevent Lesley from hearing the word, but to let me know it. She said, "Lesley talks about it as if she is still here" and I confirmed that this was consistent with her formal understanding (of the concept of death, without mentioning this word). However, we were well aware of the bereavement issues. Lesley calls out for her mother frequently. This is seen as 'challenging behaviour' and is considered annoying for the other residents and the staff themselves

This kind of expectation seems to come from:

1. Higher estimated functioning and 'deliberateness' or 'manipulation' on the part of people such as Lesley,
2. The widespread use of terms such as "having a behaviour" to refer to 'undesirable behaviour'.

This begs the question as to whom the behaviour is undesirable? Readers should note that it is rather ironic that behavioural models will contend to use 'objective' observation and recording of challenging behaviours, yet decide on whether to try to eliminate it by judging it subjectively and calling it 'undesirable'. In wanting to discourage her crying out, it seemed to us that they were travelling in the opposite direction to the actual help Lesley needed.

In the book *Meeting Emotional Needs in Intellectual Disability*, Sappok *et al* (2021) point out that people such as Lesley are engaged in an appeal when they express distress; Lesley was calling out for comfort when calling out for her mum. She was anxious and did not need to be discouraged from communicating this; instead, she needed a comforting response. Calling out for one's parent in their absence, especially when no one wants to take their place, would only be inappropriate at a much later stage in development than Lesley had reached, where the prolonged absence of caregivers is tolerable and where there are substitute intimate relationships or a partner.

Getting back to the events of the session, Lesley would talk about people and places that she missed. She spoke about these in a happy sort of way, remembering it with a warmth that contrasted with her current situation. When this happened, the staff member kept trying to let me know that this was the problem – all Lesley wants to do is go over the past. "See what she is like?" they implied in their attitude and comments

The staff would interject at intervals, saying, "Can I just tell Victoria more about that". The phrase "When we see behaviours the most is...", and

"She gets jumbled up and annoyed with herself – this is also when we see behaviours". It was as though Alessa would not let Lesley freely express herself, and I felt that no one wanted to communicate and process her grief with her.

There was an open discussion of all of her medical issues, including medication. In fact, the referral had come to me because of concerns that the staff only wanted medication changes in response to the expression of distress by Lesley. My colleagues and I felt outraged by the apparent muzzling of this vulnerable woman, and so we had taken up the referral with some urgency.

Later in the session, Alessa said, "What I don't get is, when she has been on Epilim for so long, and then taken off, that's when things changed". This was not true[3], but as if to legitimise this comment, and her disagreement with the discontinuation, she said "I've worked with Lesley for a long time". Alessa's concern was to put Lesley back on the medication, as she and her team felt that the medication made her "better". However, the reality of this regime was that Lesley was routinely prescribed medication to lower perceived distress on an ad hoc basis. In fact, to not have the option of this intervention, they considered "cruel".

A PBS plan had also been mooted. Alessa said, "I've heard about this behaviour support plan". The plan from our team from the year previously was described as "out of date", with the implied attack of neglect by our service.

In fact, they had presented asking only for medication changes and did not want a behavioural approach when they first brought the issue to the team.

Alessa then said, "Anyway, we have our own behaviour support plan". This referred to a document she had written herself, which was not actually based on a psychological understanding of Lesley, but was instead a list of responses intended to teach Lesley that staff would ignore her

3 This had been disproved the year before when a community nurse colleague had plotted incident reports against seizure reports and changes in medication. There was no apparent effect of the medication change, yet this belief in "a problem medication change" remained strong within Alessa's team. Physical explanations for distressed behaviour are very comforting for professionals and some carers because they remove the implication that their actions have been less than optimal in providing care to the person. We believe that it is very important to assess this rigorously and not simply offer an alternative theory. It is usually possible to test such ideas by time-lapse plotting. At the very least, if medication changes are indeed implicated in making things worse (or better) this will become clear by plotting it graphically.

and even leave the room if she was "obsessive". Lesley was referred to as having "a learning disability, challenging behaviour and obsessive compulsive disorder" with the apparent compulsions being to keep asking for cuddles and referring to her mum.

I really struggled with an emotion that I can only describe as a mixture of disappointment and anger, as I had developed some rapport with Alessa, but what she had done was formalise and condone, even require, emotional neglect.

The idea that one could respond to distress in terms of secure attachment caregiving had never been discussed until I brought it up. I had the workbook *Meeting emotional needs in people with severe intellectual disabilities* with me, which we encourage care teams to use and work through. This includes the model of caregiving that meets emotional needs. It includes modelling of 'four tasks of emotionally secure caregiving', tailored to the assessed level of emotional development.

Figure 3.1: Emotionally secure caregiving

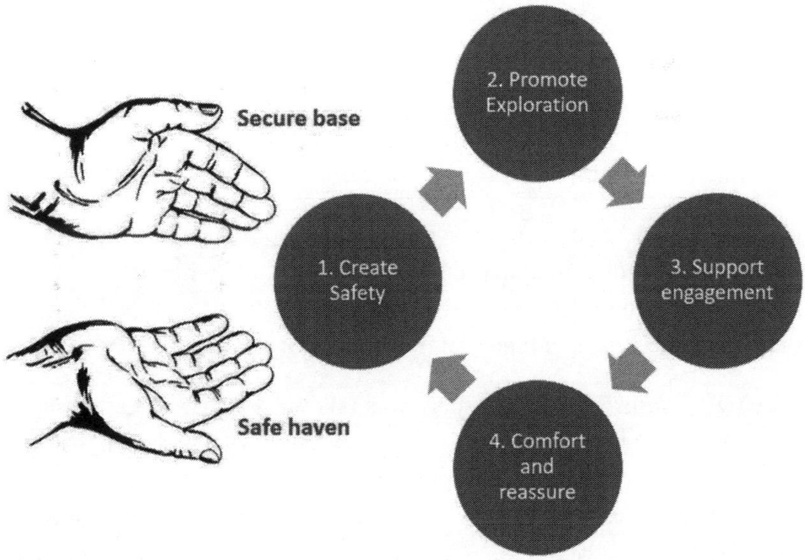

I started to show Alessa this model. She did not alter her proximity to me; there was no feeling of taking the learning offered from this model in. What I was saying had to be resisted, dismissed. This made me wonder if Lesley's needs were being dismissed in the same way, as her carers had developed a strongly avoidant pattern of caregiving. They were not physically present; they did not structure her exploration; they failed to keep her engaged in mutual activity; and her need for comfort irritated them and evoked hostility and the wish to seek powerful drugs that would dampen her emotions.

Assistance from others supports our sense of our existence, our importance to others, our sense that we will cared for when we need it. Lesley would put out her hands when she needed assistance, for example, to go to the toilet. Alessa would take her hand and put in on the sofa so she would self-propel. Lesley complied with it, but never gave up on holding her hands up in this way. It made me think of how we respond when a person early in development puts up their hands not only for assistance but for *love*.

Having worked in various care and mental health settings, I knew it did not have to be this way, but I recognised the process of emotional distancing. In my experience, a care worker forming a close bond born out of empathy and everyday kindness results in gaining a reputation of being 'soft' and somehow undermining independence. This can result in suppressing one's own caregiving impulses – responding with love – because it implies poor professional conduct. Yet at the same time, it was the main reason I went into that role. By then moving into a psychology role, I started to reconsider why forming a close bond with a person I was working with, often in some of the most vulnerable states a human being can find themselves in, receive less, not more, in the way of affection.

Eventually, when I had been there for about an hour, we talked about what would be happening later. Lunch was confirmed when Lesley said, "Are we having lunch?" Lunch, then walk, Alessa confirmed, and then I strongly felt that it was being communicated that the session had ended.

In moving towards the kitchen, there was talk of "a job" where she put out and put away the condiments each day at 5pm. Alessa asked Lesley how much she gets paid for this and she said, "A thousand pounds". I wondered, how was this a 'job' in any meaningful sense. And where were the riches? The riches were in her past and in her memory, but this is not valued in any emotional mirror offered by her care team.

A diagram that we use about avoidance in psychotherapy can show how Lesley experienced her care. She did not have a secure base, and there was no safe haven to return to, except in her mind (her calling out for her mum). Instead, she attempted to sing to herself for a while, or rock to self-soothe. Self-soothing is a telling sign of under-stimulation, but we know from the experience of severe neglect[4] that this is also a sign that the person is being deprived of love.

Figure 3.2: Avoidant attachment preventing connection

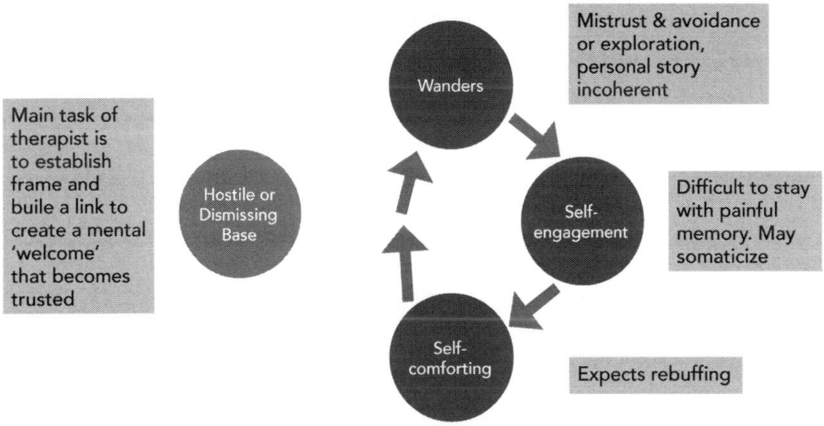

I was left feeling like I had not made a connection with the care team. We had not become attuned. Attunement refers to our ability to be aware of and respond to the emotional needs of another person, typically our children when they are babies. We were hoping to set up training for the near future, but they were only interested in a half-hearted way, as a minimal show of professionalism. Alessa asked for morning sessions, as her team would "rather get it over with in the morning", for their convenience. We were an inconvenience, a nuisance, an irritation. I did not feel warmth in our working relationship.

I happened to know another resident whom I saw in passing as I left; I had met their family. Alessa commented, "Oh really, she can't know you, as she would have said", invalidating what I knew to be true. I did not bother to contradict her. I was struck by the contrast of Alessa's delighted and joyful response to this person. But Lesley was not afforded any delight or joy, and thus she was denied yet another important aspect of love.

I would not have been surprised if, after I had left, the staff team had said to each other, "There was no point to that". By being left with this feeling,

4 The American Psychological Association have shown that neglect, such as that perpetrated on Romanian orphans prior to 1989, has devastating effects on development, that can only be partially rectified. See The lasting impact of neglect (apa.org) – www.apa.org/monitor/2014/06/neglect (accessed September 2023).

my heart sinks as I recall the woman who had no one to see her need for love, or to simply meet it.

Afterthought

We did manage to deliver a training session about Lesley's emotional development and attachment needs, with the team listening impassively, as though resentfully attending a school lesson. The only person to offer feedback was Alessa, who assured us that she offered secure caregiving, and that the four tasks of emotional security were met by the team; we did not need to observe them or visit them again.

We found out later, indirectly, that Alessa had sought contact with a psychiatrist soon after our session, asking for diazepam to be increased so that she could "calm down a bit". The psychiatrist, a rotational trainee (on placement for a set period of a few months) duly obliged, on the 'clear evidence' that Alessa's account of Lesley's "increasing disturbance" was evidence of a deteriorating 'anxiety disorder'. The disheartening element of this was not so much the increase in medication (though that did concern us), but the narratives that were used between Alessa and the psychiatrist, which comprised purely medical language and which implied the presence of mental illness. We may have caused some disturbance in this certainty that Lesley's mental illness was a fact, but even as a metaphor, it remained powerfully influential in her care. For us, she remained in a state of drugged neglect, and so our work continues to the time of writing, and remains urgent.

Chapter 4: Hannah

In your own time

> *"Vulnerability sounds like truth and feels like courage. Truth and courage aren't always comfortable, but they're never weaknesses".*
>
> Brené Brown

This chapter discusses change during long-term counselling, informed by psychoanalytic and attachment theory with Hannah, a 30-year-old woman with a mild intellectual disability. Hannah was referred by the community mental health team who had completed a course of online anxiety management on the principles of cognitive therapy. We briefly introduce the case and the point in therapy at which she decided to meet face to face. Previous sessions had been online, but Hannah had been unable to put her camera on, eventually doing so more and more until she agreed to meet face to face with Victoria Shimmens. The first face-to-face session is described. This had taken a lot of work to achieve – simply coming in to see us – and was in fact our 41st contact.

I really did not think that Hannah would attend the session as I had worked mainly to make and maintain contact with her, with working on the content of sessions being secondary to this. I had thought about disengagement a lot in supervision, and the risk of this. Being face to face removed the power to turn off the camera (whether I could see her). I was intrigued and anxious about how my personal presence, use of a mask due to COVID regulations, and body language would come across.

Hannah arrived in the reception without her chaperone. She seemed frightened and was anxiously scanning her phone. Her eyes suggested brief contact, almost as though to hold my gaze would be threatening. She mentioned that she was happy to see two members of our team who had supported her in different roles. However, I knew that it was the positivity in their working relationships and not the techniques taught that she valued. She viewed them as 'nice people' who were kind and supportive.

She followed me into the consultation rooms and I asked how she felt about coming. In. She said, "Weird, but in a good way", and, "Different, but good". I wondered if she was trying to reassure herself that this was a good thing. The therapeutic space was not yet established as safe – she needed to scan the situation first. I commented that attending for the first time is *a Strange Situation* and therefore very important. I felt proud of her in the countertransference. The power of this parental feeling seemed to suggest the absence of such pride in her family of origin, which I had gleaned from previous conversations. Saying this face-to-face seemed much more powerful. I wondered if an online relationship resonated at a more superficial level – on social media, there were often trite compliments or 'happy birthdays' from her family that I knew were not heartfelt, or at least only represented some of their feelings towards her. For example, when she achieved employment, the family focused on the short-term nature of the contract and her eventual unemployment, rather than delighting in her success.

We discussed her family. The content of the session was about having to 'pretend' a lot, change the nature of herself. She disliked having to present herself as a 'false self', that she was OK, that her father was not the alcoholic that he was. She also felt she had to pretend her mother, who had left the family home, was not distant and had not excluded her from the new family her mother had made. Hannah was expressly told that she was not to refer to her sister as "little sis". This placed her in a limbo between two families where she felt unwanted and barely tolerated by both.

She had been told to "control your anger" in situations where she had been assertive with her family in relation to being excluded. Much of what made her distressed did not seem to be her responsibility. She had, for example, confronted her father about money he had borrowed from her and not returned, to which he had responded by locking her in the bathroom. He had told her in response that he would kill himself and that it would be her fault. On another day, she had feelings of harming herself. I experienced a strong protective feeling towards her, recalling that her father had been reported for assaulting her in the past.

Both parents were reported to use alcohol, to shout at Hannah and to be unavailable or even frightening in their actions. She spoke about online sessions with me where she had been forced to relocate around the house, to prevent her parents from listening in.

Another feature of this session was that she was not able to text her friend during our allotted hour or take calls from people. The calls had seemed genuine, and I had not imposed a no-call boundary at the start of the sessions, intentionally to avoid seeming prohibitive. However, I do include this with other clients. In the first sessions, a lack of ego strength – the ability to tolerate challenges without decompensation or abreaction to therapy – seemed to risk disengagement. I realise in looking back on this first face-to-face session that she had already travelled a long way with me, although throughout the sessions I still felt that she could fail to turn up.

The task of this session was to establish a secure base/safe haven for Hannah to explore in the presence of a safe other. Most of the people in her life wanted to shut down her feelings, especially if they involved frustration, anxiety, depression or the want of love from others that was lacking. This was uncanny for Hannah. It contradicted her attachment Templates, which were intermittently available, or hostile, but never consistently loving. I noted that, after this session, she stopped trying to change the time, date and/or venue of our sessions.

Our psychodynamic formulation at this time determined that she had, in fact, no actual intrapsychic symptoms – that her presentation represented the dysfunction of her place between two unloving families. There was no evidence of anxiety, anger or other distress that was out of proportion to this situation. Indeed, a family member referred to her "not being our Hannah anymore", as she became more expressive. Insofar as she had been shouting and swearing at her family, this represented a small proportion of the swearing and shouting that took place in the family, and I traced each and every episode she described to an instance where she had received the message that she was treated differently because of her learning disability. In fact, she was expected to be quiet, demure, asexual, and completely inoffensive.

This reminds us of the point made by Sinason (2010) that there is a very particular form of requirement expected of people with intellectual disabilities, namely, that they are only allowed to live so long as they do not present with aggression or sexuality. Yet all human beings become frustrated, angry, egocentric or hopeless at times, so this façade cannot be maintained. We find that this is often at the root of referrals from families, and some professionals – that they want the psychology team to stop the client expressing what is most basic in the human psyche. That we need to be loved, and that abandonment is profoundly distressing.

This was Hannah's 41st session. I recorded a concern about her emotional and physical safety in our clinical records system. I told Hannah that she existed in my mind as an object of concern, and that I had a duty to safeguard her if this was necessary, though this would require her consent. I mentioned that she had a lot of skills and resources but needed this to be validated emotionally by someone who would act in her interests, unconditionally, until she could do this for herself.

This touches on the idea of *introjection*. Introjection is a process of 'taking in' another person so that they exist within us, which helps to form our adult personality (how we relate to others). It starts in infancy. If we experience good-enough care, what is introjected is a parent who loves us unconditionally, who sees our personal value, who can support us to explore the world, and who comforts us. To some extent, we must be frustrated and so this good-enough care is actually quite difficult to provide, as infant care is tiring, broken by work commitments, the need for the parent to care for themselves, sleep deprivation for a time, and needs to be shared with other babies.

Hannah's care was not good enough. She was not the child that was expected, and experienced a distracted, self-absorbed parent who did not respond to her needs. She therefore became self-stimulating and expected others to be unhelpful or angry with her throughout her childhood. While a therapist can replace this introjected parent to some extent, this is a serious endeavour and cannot be done quickly or easily. This is why long-term work can be needed when children have been chronically neglected, and why short-term interventions may be less effective when the person's distress is more severe and integrated into their personality than longer-term approaches (e.g Choi-Khan, 2017).

She gave me a gift; a model of a beautiful bridge structure. Hannah was at her most competent and satisfied when she had built a model she was happy with. I noted the meaning of the bridge, and indeed there seemed to be a 'psychic bridge' between our minds. While I felt some sadness that this creativity was not appreciated by her family, I was also impressed by her generosity and responsiveness to the security and exploration in the therapy. She told me she had worked for many hours on the model, which convinced me that the therapy was valuable to her.

The case is known to be successful at several levels, and indeed Hannah has gone from strength to strength, forming a very clear idea of her difficulties, and the limitations of others in her life being causal of her referral. Essentially, we have sought to remove the idea that she is intrinsically worth less than other people, a feeling that she developed from the unloving responses of family members. That she has not responded with a toxic envy of others who do not have to deal with this, because they have no learning disability and/or because their parents were unconditionally loving, is all the more remarkable. Therapists should be wary when they feel admiration for their client – it may involve idealisation, but we cannot think of Hannah without acknowledging her hard work and moral decency, her lack of vindictiveness and her dignity.

As a society that truly cares, we cannot set a number of sessions to make this kind of achievement. It has to occur at the pace of the person. It also has to be continually available, free of charge, from statutory services. We cannot expect someone like Hannah to take the insight of therapy into her life and make changes in an empowered way, especially when 'decommissioning' unsatisfactory parental figures, to comfort their inner child. Hannah could not actually hand her parents her therapeutic letter to read, even with all the changes she had achieved. People with an intellectual disability may not have an alternative support network should the family retaliate by *actual* abandonment.

This is especially relevant when a person needs to contradict important figures in their life who will have spent many years conditioning them to do what *they* wanted, and to be the person *they* want. It is no small task. To make skilled, supportive therapy difficult to access or to artificially limit its length, is at best to fall short, at worst it is to continue the neglect that affirms unlovability. We need to stand firm on this matter.

Chapter 5: Colin

Getting closer

"You never took the time to get to know me,
and your love suffered because of it".

Anonymous

Colin is in his 50s. He was referred because he had attacked a member of his care team. Colin was presented to professionals as 'forensic' and described mainly by a collection of unwanted behaviours – "punching, hitting out, kicking, shouting". No small amount of fear predated meeting Colin.

We were asked to help 'manage' his 'challenging behaviours', and to address him becoming 'over-attached' and 'obsessed with' particular members of staff. The physical abuse he had suffered on a long-stay ward was represented by how he would cower before professionals, expecting them to restrain him with painful holds (including bent wrist, arm up back). A member of his current staff who was very fond of him, Jerry, had left after Colin had hit him. On speaking to Jerry about this prior to him leaving, it was clear that Jerry really cared about Colin and had (consciously, at least) been very committed to his care. The assault appeared to have wounded Jerry so deeply that he could not bear to work with Colin anymore. There appeared to be a 'moral injury'.This chapter describes the experience of Victoria Shimmens working with him and his care team shortly after Jerry left.

I met Colin at home. As I arrived, I was welcomed but asked with some anxiety about the purpose of the visit. The person who said hello was in middle life, friendly, and open to our visit. They voiced that they did not know how he would respond to being talked to and were a little anxious about this.

I could not believe the contrast between how he had been described in his referral and his presentation; he was diminutive, looked down, and greeted me by reciting what was on the television – a *Lassie* film. He liked to watch this film over and over, a film with the theme of the lost love of a pet and the joy of reunion. He called to Lassie as though she would come through the screen to him.

I introduced myself in a light tone. I mentioned how lovely his home was, asked him what he had been doing that day, and amended a version of my role to what he might understand – to see how things were going for him. Like many clients, it was not possible to meaningfully explain the role of a psychologist straight away, though we are obliged to ensure the person knows as much as possible about our role and give consent if they can. But Colin, like many of more vulnerable people, would have found a long explanation of this confusing, even distressing. Instead, I watched for his reaction.

Initially, he did not speak to me directly, and instead pointed to pictures of staff that he had worked with. One of these he saw as "grandma". I wondered if there was a kindly grandma in his history. He did actually associate several of his favourite carers to family roles. The staff showed me his visual planner (a picture calendar) and how he had been to Bradford FC football ground.

He gestured for me to come into his room, then put his hands up to make me take care. Colin had created a game where he had attached some string to the top of his bedroom door. His care team were invited to shimmy around this before entering his room. Certain objects were not to be moved, for example, his most recent Bradford FC drawings and a trophy he had made. I noted that he was very creative within his own interests.

He shouted for two members of his care team, Margo and John, to come in and join us. They then engaged in a rehearsed, warm and affectionate to-and-fro. He said he would hide Margo's slippers and she said, "You will not mind". I noticed that they brought their slippers to respectfully care for his flooring. This interchange, though repetitive, appeared to be enjoyed by everyone.

Colin has an imaginary friend whom he calls 'Bertie'. We were invited to sit on the floor together. Margo and John asked Colin to show me what he does when he "feels worried", as they put it. He showed me the stress ball that he squeezes, then lay back doing his "breathing techniques" where he would hold his chest and breathe. This wasn't actually slow, deep breathing that would have a calming effect. I felt it was actually closer to hyperventilating, which increases distress. He started to cry and referred to "telling Bertie", which I took to mean he could not process painful feelings directly in this way. I reassured him by laying next to him and asking to hold his hand. Colin asked Margo lay down on the other side, and I mentioned that he wouldn't feel upset for long and that he would be OK. I modelled this on the fourth task of secure caregiving which is derived from attachment theory (see Chapter 3 & Figure 3.1).

It struck me that this was not meaningful to him, it was to please them, to be a performance of the "good boy". As can be seen in Figure 5.1, his emotional development is not consistent with the self-sufficient use of 'arousal management' techniques. The comfort he required was the reassurance of love – deep, enduring love in a family-style environment. There was to be no real comfort in slowing down his breathing or squeezing a piece of rubber (in the first individuation stage, normally seen at the 18-month to three-year level, comforting is physical-focused rather than mental, with eye contact, supportive tones and reassuring words that do not have to be formally understood in language. The person is not expected to be able to self-soothe at this stage.)

We often have a feeling that 'techniques' are attempted when our clients are distressed and causing discomfort in others. It is as though Colin's care team felt the need to "do something", something that could be acted for me, for me to approve of. I wondered why it is not OK to simply be unsure what to do, and instead to do nothing, but witness distress, reassure the person, and wait for the feeling to evolve into something that is easier to bear. It seemed shameful in some way, if they didn't have the stress ball or the breathing technique.

What lay beneath the tears was the death of his dad. It turns out that Colin's dad was a lifelong Bradford Football Club supporter. In fact, the main concern of the staff was what to do if he spoke of his dad, and if they were "doing enough". On previous visits by professionals, they would discuss "techniques", using feeling cards and objects of reference, to make this into a 'game' so that he could talk about the happier memories. There was something about these discussions that had struck me as 'sanitising' the session and creating a kind of professional credibility, something substantial.

But the techniques missed the point. The difficulty was not necessarily with Colin. It was his carers who were unsure, guilty, anxious. They needed a framework for their own feelings. To know that they were providing the kind of care that would help him to experience his losses without this becoming a terrible, unremitting misery. In this, there must be some capacity to stay with sorrow and sadness. As it happened, one member of staff then tentatively volunteered that, “I lost my mam. I know what it is like. How hard it is. And I know my dad and your dad would want us to remember them. I think they might be together in heaven.” This idea was full of empathy and kindness[5].

It’s important to say that, at this time, the use of this language of love and loss was felt to be taboo when professionals were visiting. Something like relief came over our working relationship when they realised that we wanted to talk using these terms, to see them as loved and loving towards their ‘client’. While there can be no doubt that some of the formal therapeutic techniques such as mindfulness or breathing techniques are helpful for some people, these must be delivered within a substantial relationship where there is a secure attachment. Without a secure base and safe haven, there can be no independence.

We spent further sessions working ‘by proxy’ with Colin’s care team. I visited again, to observe them working with him. We conversed with them, and in the process they stopped seeing his actions as a kind of chess game in which he would make moves to meet some selfish end. We pointed up the warmth they already showed him. Together with them, we realised that no one had ever been so close to him. They would encourage him to explore his world and would comfort him when he was anxious. They realised that their delight in things like shopping or a visit to a restaurant was integral to his future. They were no longer imagining that he would visit the restaurant alone a year hence. Instead, they accepted that this was it; they would be in an affectionate bond for as long as they were his caregivers. This commitment was more than enough to deal with Colin’s anxieties and occasional acts of frustration.

Closeness involves risk; risk of being hurt and of eventual grief. Closeness is absolutely necessary, however, to truly understand a person like Colin. This was also true of our relationship with the care team. They trusted that we cared, would help them explore, provide a framework for understanding, and comfort them when they were sad or anxious about him.

Everyone working with people who have intellectual disabilities should get closer to those they are trying to help.

5 The understanding of death in people with significant intellectual disabilities is not always straightforward. Colin did not have a formal understanding of death except that he would not see his father and that it was final. I was never clear on whether he thought his father still existed spiritually. In this context, the idea of “being in heaven” was not in any clear relation to Colin’s beliefs. We took the view that the idea was helpful, given that the context was his carer using the idea to provide comfort.

References

Choi-Kain LW, Finch EF, Masland SR, Jenkins JA & Unruh BT (2017) What works in the treatment of borderline personality disorder. *Current Behavioral Neuroscience Reports*, **4**, 1, 21–30.

Chapter 6: Renata

Nobody loves me, and neither do I

This chapter is about Renata, whose history is a litany of abuse and unforgivable neglect by care services. Renata has been seeing Allan for psychological therapy for several years. We have tried to learn from her and are in awe of her dignity in the face of such indifference and unwarranted contempt towards her.

Renata had been referred in her late 40s, the daughter of a traveller family living in the north east of England. The family had given up their wagons for council houses when she was an infant, but there was still a strong tradition of buying and selling horses by way of cash and handshake. She lived on her own in a small flat overlooking a small common that would often be home to horses in an otherwise urban environment. It was only after several overdoses and presentations to the local emergency department that she was considered as perhaps having some kind of intellectual disability. When she was finally assessed, our team was shocked to find that, despite going to a special school in the 1970s, she had never formally been diagnosed.

Renata's life was hard from the start. She had a stroke when she was a baby, leaving her with an obvious facial disfigurement that marked her out for protracted and often serious bullying. She remembered her parents openly favouring her siblings and allowing them to call her "the spacca" (a derogatory term derived from the word 'spastic'). She was locked in a room without a window for several hours a day while her parents drank. There was enough to eat, but there was no overt expression of affection for Renata, unlike her brothers who were cuddled and praised, especially for "cleverness". Perhaps picking up on her unwelcome status in the family, when she was seven years old, her brothers decided to see if she would survive being pushed down the stairs. She did, but she has suffered from double vision and headaches ever since the fall.

After school, Renata got a job in a bar for a while, but could not do this safely, and was repeatedly exposed to unwanted sexual activity. She was eventually raped and then driven in the back of a car into the countryside, fully expecting to be killed. She was dumped in the open with no way of getting home and had to walk to a nearby house and ask for help. No one was ever arrested or convicted for these crimes.

Renata had one meaningful relationship as a young adult, and for a time found some contentment with Barry, who had known her via a friendship group. He was affectionate, attentive and sensitive, calling her "my little miracle". However, after a year of real love and a stable home life, Barry developed a serious illness and died very suddenly. While she was grieving, local criminals threatened Renata for money which they claimed Barry had owed them.

When finally offered psychotherapy at the age of 46, Renata was confused. It was as though kindness or the offer of a conversation was entirely new to her. She said, "I am the lost one, the black sheep. Why would you want to help me?" She reported low mood and self-diagnosed depression. She blamed herself and had no self-esteem. She had lost any dignity she may have had and could not see any reason for carrying on.

A typical session with Renata in her third year of seeing me occurred as follows. She was, as usual, right on time. She would come in and say, "Hello Dr Allan", with warmth and kindness, searching for reciprocation on my face, and lighting up when I replied. On occasion, I would break the 'frame' of psychotherapy by offering her a coffee. She responded to this as though it was the act of ultimate kindness, with the broadest of smiles and "Two sugars, like you know".

Renata would almost always start a session by saying, "I haven't been very good". There would follow a discussion of a relatively minor issue – a bureaucratic glitch with her benefits, or a minor disagreement about her support hours with her care provider. But this was only the opening to the underlying issue of a fundamental desolation in her mind, a lack of the ability to accept the positive regard of her therapist and see within this her basic human value. This was all the more painful for me to witness because I knew that, by any objective standard, Renata was a moral, decent person who would lay down her life to prevent a child or a vulnerable person from being harmed.

"I am lost. I am the black sheep."

The phrase was never far away. She believed it irrespective of the evidence. Irrespective of the affection poured upon her from her care team, who would jostle their rotas to work with her, she continued to believe that she was unworthy of living. This was almost comfortingly familiar and kept her in some form of – rejected – relationship with her family. In particular, Renata's mother expected her to visit her every day, collect medication for her, and carry out other tasks. At the same time, she was not invited to family occasions. This was not in the time of the pandemic. This was simply how the family saw her – as a non-member of their family.

There were exceptions. There was a nephew who could not bear Renata to be left out and made it a point of principle to regularly include her in birthdays, Easter and Christmas family events. Renata was most happy when with this nephew's sons, and with the unconditional acceptance of young children, they would climb on top of her and provide her with the kind of love that she had never received herself as a child. She often remarked that the thought of seeing them hurt was the thing that kept her from suicide.

As we talked over many months, and eventually years, Renata came to accept at a formal, rational level that she had some worth, and she changed her view that professionals only showed an interest for financial gain. She recognised that some were actually fond of her. However, she was very resistant to thinking about the kind of abuse that Miller (1985) described as small, everyday, but significant punishments that have lifelong effects on our self-esteem and our ability to afford ourselves any kindness or leeway when we err. Talking to Renata was a continual reminder of the immense and unwavering loyalty that children have to their parents, no matter how poor they seem as parents to others looking in.

Renata told me about her regular visits to her father, who was terminally ill, but would not tell her what was wrong with him. She told me that she could not tell her father about her mental health because he would become instantly enraged and shout, "What about me?!" She feared him but kept going back for more. She was excluded from family events if her father was there. She would ask me rhetorically, "Am I not family?", and noted bitterly that she was told she could not attend a wedding because it was "family only". Her reasoning about why she bothered to have this daily contact was, "It's me dad, at the end of the day", when many people in her life, including her care team, advised her to break contact.

As often happened in sessions, discussing this would lead to Renata talking about what she would do if her sessions ever came to an end. She would kill herself, because she is a "waste of space". That she placed the blame on the professionals around her was thinly veiled, but she denied it when I would suggest that this is actually rather demanding and unfair. In fact, it created the feelings in my psyche that her family had for her; you are manipulative and demanding, and I want to be rid of you. Overcoming this impulse to discharge the case and blaming the lack of progress with her depression on her manipulative threats had required a lot of clinical supervision. I eventually connected to the fact that long-term work was needed, because she could not safely separate and live as an adult without feeling abandoned and terrified.

However, these comments did not lead to any hopelessness about the therapy; at least, at a conscious level. Instead, after about two years of therapy, Renata would threaten to kill herself, "Because there is no point being here", but then say, "Don't worry, I won't do anything stupid", and then, imply that, "It is only because of you that I am alive". This huge overvaluing of the therapist was incredibly seductive, an invitation to idealisation. But it did not reduce her anxiety or fear of being lost to others. Soon after making such comments about the high value of the therapist, she would offer some expression of suspicion that I was secretly planning her discharge. She needed to feel that she was not too depressed to be an out-patient, but also dangerous enough to herself to need therapy forever. I was reminded of a paper by Barth (2009) who described both the *idealisation* of parents – the insistence that they were wonderful in the presence of ample evidence to the contrary; and *parent-blaming*, which itself can ward off deeper, more conflicted feelings. Barth noted that psychotherapists may consider negative feelings about parents to be more 'real' than positive emotions, but this can help the person avoid the painful understanding of the parents' own sorrows and deprivations. Therapists can easily identify with the parent-blaming to support their client, but this is not actually helpful, because it involves distortion. In reality, no one is fully evil, or fully good. As young children, we quickly flit between these positions when looking at our parents, depending on how they thwart or satisfy us. The ability to 'flit' from "I hate you" to "I love you" without connecting to the contradiction is called splitting, and this remains a defence that is deployed in times of threat or stress when we are older. In some, such thinking actually dominates, usually because their childhood was particularly awful.

When I mentioned to Renata that therapy could not provide what her parents should have given her, she would become extremely sad, even tearful. She would say, "At the end of the day, it's me mam and dad". This wasn't logical – there was little in her descriptions of her childhood care that was affectionate and much that was rejecting, favouring her siblings, and there were even overt wishes that she did not exist or had died in childhood. But what alternative do children have when the only adults available to them cannot love them properly? The anger and idealisation that should fall apart in the face of truly loving parents – who keep their children safe, help them explore, stay attuned to their emotions, and comfort them in times of distress or pain – remains and crystalises in the personality. We have come to consider this as *loyalty to the parental object*[6]. The expectation that negative experiences of parental care would lead to a fundamental lack of respect for their parenting instead becomes a compulsive seeking for the love that the person 'knows' is 'really there'. Renata would say, "I know they loved me, they just didn't show it". Her deepest fear was being told not to return, for that meant abandonment and death. Her comments about suicide were an appeal – to see love and value in another person's eyes. She had instead received what Miller (1985) calls *poisonous pegagogy* – being taught how to live via repeated abuses.

Therapy was therefore strange, disloyal and frightening for Renata. "No one loves me. And neither do I", she said.

It would take years before she could even recall and name all of the traumas that had been visited upon her. Our own relationship developed from an idealised saviour–persecuted victim dynamic to a more limited partnership. Conversations did not 'save' Renata anymore; they were helpful, but not transformative; she started to accept that her father could never become what she wanted. She would have to love herself. We often discussed the metaphor of the *inner child*. The inner child can be a very useful metaphor when clients are cruel to themselves. They tend to value children's well-being and become upset, or even have a trauma response (freezing, flashbacks, extreme emotion, desperate escape behaviours) when they see children being maltreated. They will voice moral behaviours and the wish to correct the parents and have the child treated better. It can be both useful and shocking for clients to conceptualise themselves

6 Melanie Klein proposed the idea of 'objects', which are the mental representations of other people in our minds. We are necessarily limited in our understanding of others – in one sense, we only know others as the ideas we have of them, which are distorted by our own desires, fears, wishes and other unconscious feelings. This can have huge effects on our ability to have relationships with others, if the distortions prevent any true connection with other people.

as having an inner child and realise how cruel they have been behaving to that child, in a way that they would never be to other children; to think of one's inner five-year-old, and how we would comfort them, tell them it was never their fault, and commit to loving and protecting them. To realise that one has kept doing the abuse to one's own inner child, by internalising it, is a shock, but it can be transformative.

In Renata's case, this finally mobilised her to be kinder to herself. She began to say, "Sometimes I feel like I am worth something". This was not straightforward or felt without the accompanying feeling that she was somehow wrong about this. It was as though to value herself would upset someone who would then attack her. I suggested that she should think of herself ("that little girl", she called her) as a strong adult who is finally loving her little self in the way she deserves.

Yet, Renata found changing her actual behaviour towards her family much more difficult than thinking about it. She would have to challenge their criticism of her and imply that they had actually caused some of her distress. Given that they were already ambivalent towards her, this felt like risking that they would simply cut her off completely, leaving her feeling totally abandoned. An abandoned inner child is an unbearable feeling, and Renata would continue to say, "At the end of the day, it's my family". This loyalty to the parental object, however bad the maltreatment, is something we repeatedly experience in our work.

A key idea in psychodynamic approaches is that of *transference*. This involves feelings that belong in the family of origin being projected onto the therapist. That is to say, that what was felt about the parents is also felt about the therapist, even though the therapist may not have those characteristics. For example, as the therapist points out that the time has come to an end and the session must stop, the person may perceive that they are being rebuffed or pushed out, as this was their experience as a child.

Another feature of this phenomenon is *countertransference*. This refers to the feelings the therapist receives when transference is active. These can be understood as unhelpful or even mixed up with the personal feelings of the therapist themselves, which is to be avoided[7]. However, where this

---

7 Hence the insistence in psychodynamic therapy on personal therapy for professional practitioners. It is vitally important that the therapy meets the needs of the person seeking help and does not simply support the emotional life and satisfactions of the professional.

confusion does not arise (hopefully, most of the time), the therapist can see these emotional responses as a source of information that can become useful in supporting the client.

I often felt that Renata needed to be looked after and made safe[8]. Trust was a key issue, and while she was very complimentary about the therapy, I always felt accused of abandonment and dereliction of care. This conversation was very hard for Renata to have directly with her family. They seemed to have an uncanny sense of any such conversation starting, and become aggressive to ward it off, telling her to leave, or leaving themselves, in a hostile manner.

In the end, Renata did acknowledge that her family were never going to offer what she needed. She drank alcohol even though it began to badly affect her health, and this only lessened when she decided that her care team were now her family of choice. Again, at times of stress this would become a paranoia, e.g. in comments like, "You only care because you are paid". However, in general, she was becoming sadder and more resolved, and less angry and suicidal. Her drinking became moderate, and at times experienced as pointless, and she began to look forward to her sessions as a source of care. This will eventually become a matter of social care, rather than a therapeutic intervention, because she is unlikely to garner enough internal resources to live a solitary life.

It is still ongoing work for Renata. What comes with caring for her inner child is the loss of any hope that her parents will ever love her the way she wants. She has yet to forgive them, and may never do so completely. As her father approaches the end of his life, I cannot predict with certainty that she will be okay, but I am more hopeful that she will feel okay enough not to blame herself or give up on life after he has gone. The ambivalence is not extreme anymore; they are not wonderful or evil; instead, what remains is somewhere between a painful longing and awareness that her childhood can only partially be healed. She still wants their love, even when it has never been on offer.

---

8 The feeling of wanting to look after Renata was very strong and on several occasions I wanted to act on her behalf. I literally "identified" with her "projection" of a loving father, and almost acted as though that was my role. Emotional communication of this type – that actually involves a feeling that pushes a therapist to act beyond their role – can be seen as **projective identification**. The prime example of this is when a young child cries in distress. We become distressed ourselves and begin to imagine how to react to decrease the distress. However, this cannot predominate as we get older, as wider society would not protect us unconditionally, like our parents do; so we have to "hold" what we would otherwise project and form ideas that we can communicate in words, not distressing cries or desperate acts.

References

Barth FD (2010) Frozen in Time: idealisation and parent-blaming in the therapeutic process. *Clinical Social Work Journal*, **38** 331-340.

Miller A (1985) *The Drama of Being a Child: the Search for the True Self.* London: Virago.

Chapter 7: Leonard

They don't feel that

"Indifference, to me, is the epitome of evil".

Elie Weisel

Leonard is an 18-year-old man who does not communicate using spoken language, although he does vocalise. He attends a day service five times a week. Victoria Shimmens was asked to see him because he has been reported to become angry when anyone said "no" or to "stop". This coincided with the lockdown period due to COVID. This is a brief account of the first visit to meet him at his day service.

I arrived at the day service and greeted the receptionist. She asked if we knew where we were going and when I confirmed that I did, she waved us through casually. Making our way down the corridor, other people who came to the centre would approach, excited by the arrival of a new person. Leonard was sitting watching online videos on a large screen. This was his scheduled activity for the whole of the observation. I sat down beside him, made eye contact and said, "Hi".

The first thing said to me was by Donald, his care worker, who said "You know he is non-verbal, yeah?" without looking at or acknowledging Leonard. It became immediately clear that, while Donald was keen to speak with me, he was implying that I could not interact with Leonard until he had had a two-way conversation with me first, despite my attempt to position my body towards Leonard. Leonard reached for Donald's hand, to take the computer mouse and change which video was on. It was clearly irritating Donald that Leonard would not sit through an entire video.

The process of offering the video was not an interactive process. They would silently type in a search item to locate a video they thought he might like, then look at him impassively to see if he indicated that he was happy with this. He would take his hand away from the mouse if he liked what was on offer. I noticed the lack of any joy or mutuality in the interaction. I felt the strong urge to intervene, to speak to Leonard about his video choices, to add the element of emotional connection. It should be borne in mind that this was when full personal protective equipment was required, and I was dressed in a full apron, with surgical gloves and a mask, making connection even less likely.

At this point, Donald announced how long he had worked with Leonard. He told me that things were very different because of COVID. He asked if I wanted to go through any paperwork. When I asked what happened before COVID, he said that he could not remember, then started to ask about my professional background, and how long I worked with the team. I answered briefly. Donald said that if I didn't want to review paperwork, and there was "nothing else", then he was going to check his emails. He got up and went to the other side of the room and sat with his back to Leonard and me.

Just then, a previous key worker, Mel, who had worked with Leonard before, walked into the room. She was supporting another person but made a point of coming across to speak to Leonard. She made eye contact with him at the level where he was sitting and said, "Hello, Lenny". His face lit up with a huge smile. She turned to me and said, "I miss him so much. They moved me because of the pandemic. I can't work out why exactly. All the shifts got moved around." She said, "It must be so confusing for the clients. It must be scary because we don't know how to explain the changes in staff." Leonard was holding her hands, smiling and looking at her. As she discussed the difficulties, directing this to me, he continued to watch where she was looking.

She had to go back to the client she was with. She said, "See you soon, bonny lad". She walked out into the next room. Leonard clapped a little while she was there, then went back to his video. What struck me was that Donald, who continued to ignore Leonard, seemed to find the intrusion irritating, and that the showing of emotion by Leonard was something to be discouraged. Donald appeared to blame Mel's coming in to speak to Leonard for the fact that Leonard now indicated that he wanted interaction. Donald got up, came over, sighed, and said in a resigned tone, "What do you want on now?", meaning, "What video can I put on that will quiet you?" But the question was laden with unconscious meaning. In one way, it seemed like the easiest question in the world to answer – he wanted Mel. Leonard rose and took Donald's hand in an invitation to dance. Donald said to me, "This is what he does, sometimes". Leonard extended his arms and rocked, happily, from side to side to the music that he had activated on his video screen.

In a short time, Donald lost interest and terminated the activity. He dropped his hands, saying “Enough”, and walked back to his seat. It later transpired that speech and language therapists could build strongly on this kind of initiation by Leonard, extending this into meaningful interaction that built his connection. Donald was no longer a part of the care team by then, but even at the time I had a pang of sadness at the lost opportunity.

As the session continued, I noted that Donald was not providing sufficient exploration or engagement with Leonard. Not only this, but he was unwelcoming of Leonard’s approaches. Nor could he see or appreciate the value of the kind of connection that Mel had offered. This was making Leonard aggressive in response to approaches to complete his personal care, because of the mixed message that he was unwelcome to approach, to seek help. Any aggression could therefore be seen as internalising Avoidant Attachment.

When my colleague with whom I had visited came in and told us that her interview was over, Donald’s colleague, who she had been interviewing, said she would photocopy some incident sheets and left to do this.

My colleague said care at this day service seems to be about nothing but personal care and getting into cars to go home. I said, “Also, let’s consider that there has been disruption to his routine and changes in his care staff”. I said, “He is obviously going to miss them”. Donald’s response was, “They don’t feel that”.

I felt such a chill at this comment, not only in relation to who ‘they’ were – a form of extreme othering, but in the breath-taking ease with which he could deny feelings of loss and the profound effect this may have had on Leonard, fully justified in offering only cold company and a large TV.

In leaving Leonard, I was determined to improve the understanding of his situation. The behavioural assessment did not help Leonard; it simply caused his care team to become wary around his personal care. We linked with speech and language therapy colleagues to develop the Intensive Interaction approach with Leonard.

Intensive Interaction[9], as defined by the British Institute of Learning Disabilities, is a practical approach to interacting with people with learning disabilities who do not find it easy to communicate or be social. The approach helps the person and their communication partners to relate better to each other and enjoy each other's company more. It helps them develop their communication abilities. In Intensive Interaction, the carer, support worker, speech and language therapist or teacher works on being a better communication partner and so supports the person with learning disabilities to develop confidence and competence as a communicator.

Intensive Interaction is a fun process. The communication partner is guided by what we know about how communication ordinarily develops for young children. They apply this knowledge in a way that is sensitive and respectful to the person with a learning disability, whatever their age. By showing that attunement, following the person's lead, and providinga one-to-one approach, intensive interaction provides completely secure caregiving that is entirely consistent with attachment theory principles. In this case, the outcome of working in this way proved its value to Leonard. Scientific Momentary Time Sampling (the moment to moment coding of observed actions over a time period of 60 minutes) showed a threefold increase in Leonard's interaction in any given hour when this approach was followed, with zero 'challenging behaviour' recorded during intensive interaction sessions

We soak up both verbal and non-verbal messages from those around us. Leonard watched others, listened to them, and turned towards them. His speech therapist and those who she managed to convince to follow the approach, took the opportunities that Leonard was offering them, to connect to him. Part of this was to focus *on just being with him* as the essential part of the work – the very essence of his care. It is not clear if this transformative approach really penetrated his care team, as the indifference to his need for love because of his intellectual disability was very deeply ingrained. Moreover, it probably contradicted some of the avoidant caregiving impulses of some members of staff, who would simply then avoid the client and their training, and the support of the speech therapist.

We remain in touch with Leonard. We continue to struggle with our ambivalence to his care team, and its institutional coldness which has not gone away.

9 For more information, access the bild.org.uk website

Chapter 8: LeBron

It's like a prison

> *"To restore the human subject at the centre – the suffering, afflicted, fighting human subject – we must deepen a case history to a narrative or tale; only then do we have a 'who' as well as a 'what'."*
>
> Oliver Sacks, *The Man Who Mistook His Wife for a Hat*

LeBron is a 20-year-old man with Afro-Caribbean heritage who has a severe intellectual disability. He suffered a haemorrhagic stroke when he was a baby. Curiously, LeBron had received a lot of assessment by the statutory services, but there was still no clear understanding of why he would become suddenly very distressed and attack those around him, overreacting to minor frustrations, which would often lead to someone getting hurt, often LeBron himself. Such was the concern that he lived on a hospital ward. This chapter describes a joint visit by Victoria Shimmens to a private Assessment and Treatment Ward he was detained within on a countryside campus.

I attended the ward visit with a colleague, Roy, an occupational therapist. Roy was engaged in a regular course of activities that LeBron found interesting and useful. The idea was to carry out an observation of this intervention to compare it to times when LeBron was expected to occupy himself. This was a behavioural methodology called 'interval time sampling', for which I would code the behaviour of the colleague and LeBron's response to this in both conditions. We intended to 'prove' that this way of working with LeBron would lead to the hospital staff copying this practice.

We got there and had to wait in reception. We waited 15 minutes before our arrival time. Then a healthcare assistant came out and handed us an alarm key and said, "I forgot to get you a spare key, here's mine", and then gestured in LeBron's direction to say, "He's over there". As we entered, LeBron was on one side of the room covered in a weighted blanket while his staff sat on chairs on the other side of the room, about three metres from him in order to block the doorway. This was official, legal *segregation* that was officially judged to be due to his mental health under the Mental

Health Act 1983, and in his best interests. Without addressing LeBron, one of the staff turned to us and said, "He's had a bad night", as though to justify why they were not interacting with him.

They asked if we were in a rush, as though to say he would not engage in the session. They approached and asked who we were and what our roles were. The irony of this is that my colleague was a regular visitor and should have been well known, whereas when visited, agency staff were often new and less known to LeBron. LeBron introduced us to his care team, saying, "These are [organisation name] transition staff". This refers to the intention, which he was made aware of regularly, that he was not welcome to stay in the hospital long-term and was kept there because of his behaviour.

LeBron said, "What are we doing today?" and rose from his 'Sensit' chair (a chair with a massaging function) to the table for his session with Roy. Roy said, "We are going to make some food", to which LeBron sat up and smiled. He remembered that Roy had said this on a recent visit, and he always enjoyed the sessions with him.

I had completed a lot of joint work with Roy, who was a skilled, upbeat and lively person who could usually engender delight in many people he worked with. LeBron started to work with him, but I could not be the 'uninterested observer' with LeBron, which my behavioural training required. I knew that this would be too frightening and perhaps remind LeBron of professionals who had been involved in traumatic times in his early life, such as when he had been detained and taken to hospital, and when he had been arrested and kept overnight in a cell. He kept looking over at me, as if to check that I was not critical of him. I would answer him when he asked me something. Roy had a strong relationship with LeBron, and in 18 months of working with him, had never been assaulted, nor had to end a session because of self-harm. This contrasted with the regular incident reports from the ward staff, who were frequently assaulted to the point where LeBron was restrained by up to five members of staff at a time. It was known that this was more likely when staff did not know him well, yet the way the ward was organised meant that he could work with almost 30 staff in any one day.

LeBron maintained very good interaction with Roy while I stood observing, although answering LeBron when he wanted to talk to me. He was, in fact, a reasonable conversationalist, and talked on many subjects, from the government to his family to his holidays as a child.

Roy and LeBron spoke of the successful cooking they had done in the last session. LeBron said warmly, “I want to do that”, and then mentioned a cookie he had the day before. During this interaction with us, he tried to ask his care team to join the conversation. However, they would respond by speaking to each other, for example, by saying, “There are no cookies for him today, they have all gone”.

It struck me that the baking task had so much symbolism – an activity to make an enjoyable food that can be shared – and made in a shared way, with Roy. But without Roy, the cookies are not available. The cookies could almost be love. Roy wants to make LeBron feel safe, to make something lovely, to join LeBron in making them and the joy of handing them out, and to provide this consistently, without frustrating him with intermittence, or unavailability. Consequently, Roy was a hugely positive influence on LeBron. It suddenly struck me that it was not what Roy did in the activity, but what he did in his relationship with LeBron, that made all the difference. He loved LeBron, but this had to be voiced as “I love working with LeBron”. The baking was just a prop.

None of this was available from the ward staff. They watched, fearfully. They offered nothing of what Roy could offer – engagement, support, delight and true comfort for his anxieties. They offered only ‘safe physical handling’ with a constant danger of them enjoying the restraint and isolating LeBron as a kind of revenge for what they saw as unpredictable, unwarranted, premeditated violence. I felt that they hated him, but hid this behind a professional veneer, which was sometimes very thin. For example, one staff member commented when they saw LeBron self-harming, by saying, “Well, the only one you’re hurting is yourself; eventually you will learn, or you won’t, no skin off my nose”.

When Roy left the room momentarily to seek further equipment for baking, the staff stepped further back from LeBron. He spoke about missing the patients after he left, but not really missing the staff – but then, in a revealing moment, asked them if they would visit him. One of them snorted, “Only if I have to”.

Suddenly there was a changeover of staff. His two assigned people to this point got up and walked off. They did not say goodbye. Two new people sat down in their seats. I noted that they did not know me either, but this time they did not even ask why I was there. LeBron seemed to be trying to distract himself from the changeover by putting on a new video game. While all of this was going on, two members of 'therapeutic' and 'activities' staff from the ward briefly entered his room. LeBron asked each of these what he would be doing that day. They referred to future activities later in the day, vaguely, but also interacted with the care staff who said, "Well, he's been unsettled". I suspected that there would be relief if they could cancel their planned interactions with LeBron. I also felt that the ignoring of the strangeness of my observation and the way professionals spoke or ignored each other created an uncanniness to the situation, a kind of pervasive, mild embarrassment, that one did not feel quite welcome, that one did not 'belong' here. I felt desperate for the session to end, but I knew that LeBron also wanted to escape.

The two different staff members had now sat down in the distant seating arrangement while Roy returned to begin the baking activity. LeBron tried to start a conversation with them, to which they replied with a cringe-worthy, "Yes, sir", to be humorous. Again, in response to requests from him, such as going out, they spoke to each other in response and tended to ignore him or answer him in a cursory way which did not seem fully engaged, or even respectful.

Roy began to work with LeBron on the baking task in earnest. Despite the language of 'hyperactivity' that was often applied to him, he worked with Roy for more than 90 minutes. His only moment of distress was to express concern for another patient shouting "Get me out of here!" I wondered where any insanity lay – with the 'mental and behavioural problems' of the patients, or in the fact that they were locked together in a place they could not escape, without any love. A place of fear, anger, control and containment. The only response to his concern for the other patient was for the staff to close the door, emphasising his segregation even more.

Eventually, Roy went to put the baking in the oven, at which time LeBron tried again to interact with his care team. They were talking to each other, looking at personal devices, and looking towards another patient who was in some distress. I could not bear it. I responded to some of his questions so that he would feel that at least someone was listening to him. He then tried to introduce me to those who were supposed to be his close support team. They ignored him.

When Roy returned, he engaged LeBron in a singalong. He engaged well and Roy began to ask the staff to join in. They said they were unable to. Roy then joined LeBron in a sports-based video game, and via his interest in this game, conversed with him about football. LeBron responded positively, and then began to admit to some more vulnerable aspects of himself; that he likes female staff to do his shoelaces up, that there are staff he would like to work with him, but that he has no control over this. He even explained how one person would "Run away, out of the room" if he even stands up. At points, LeBron seemed amused by this, but I could see that it was tragic. He had a kind of power at that moment, but it was a very powerless life.

Roy left the room to retrieve the baking. I noticed that if food was wanted, LeBron would ask for it, and a member of staff would retrieve it and put it in front of him. I wondered why he was not allowed to get the food himself. Then, suddenly and unexpectedly, a man walked in without uniform, and without speaking to anyone else, sat down beside LeBron, and began to interact with him. Lebron said, "Hello!" excitedly as he came in. There was no introduction to me or the hospital staff, and this felt extremely strange and intrusive. I later found out that this man was part of a team that would work with LeBron once he left the hospital. It made me wonder how random the arrivals and disappearances of staff must seem to LeBron – that other people were strange, unpredictable and often treated each other strangely, e.g., by ignoring each other.

Then a senior member of the hospital staff came into the room. The man who had entered suddenly became quiet. She asked LeBron about his day. LeBron asked if he was 'being told off' and the person responded, "I cannot be bothered to tell you off today, so you better be good today, you better be a good lad".

LeBron then spoke of writing a list and the staff member came closer to LeBron and wrote this for him and left saying they would see to this. All staff in the room proceeded to speak of an incident which had previously occurred and seemed to be ongoing, which had been heard by LeBron and those in his room. LeBron continued to actively seek social interaction with staff using their first and surnames. They did not respond, and eventually LeBron appeared to disengage. On further attempting to make a joke with staff about 'smelly feet' and changing shoes, staff members did engage and laughed with LeBron.

Roy returned with the baking, praising LeBron for how well they had come out, and LeBron proceeded to eat some of his handiwork. LeBron spoke of being very, very tired now and when asked by Roy what he was doing this afternoon, LeBron replied "Just chilling". LeBron was tentatively approached by a therapist from the hospital who asked him to join an exercise session later. He said that he didn't fancy it, to which they responded, "OK then another time", and quickly exited the situation.

Roy and I said our goodbyes to LeBron, and we were approached by the 'activities' staff. They expressed concerns about vague 'issues' and 'waiting times' as reasons why the kind of work Roy did was not part of a structured programme. They said that he "predominantly self-occupies". Roy disagreed with them. This appeared to create awkwardness as we left, and we resolved to take our concerns about the approach of the hospital staff further on our return to base.

On leaving, no management or staff were available to speak with us. I contacted the service manager upon arriving back to the community base setting to report immediately what was observed today. After telling her everything about the visit, I went to a quiet area and sat down. I found myself in tears after this session. Despite several years in the care sector and working in a community learning disabilities team, I had never seen people with an intellectual disability in such a locked, impersonal environment, who were 'un-cared for' by people who hardly knew them, who changed over every two hours, and who simply watched and waited for problems. They did not understand – did not want to understand – that LeBron's developmental level required a much more active approach, even when laid out in front of them by Roy.

LeBron continues to be understood not as someone who needs a warm, engaging and structured approach to his life, but instead as a man who is unpredictable, violent and manipulative. His current care team are more concerned with training in physical restraint and applying body armour than with supporting, listening and understanding. He is still expected to occupy himself, to tolerate unpredictable responses from others, and even to be let down by his family and visitors, who promise to visit him or to take him on an enjoyable trip. There is a continuing belief that LeBron needs to be locked up, restrained, feared and denied control of his own life. This exists both in the spoken conversations about him and in the narratives that appear in his clinical records, the medicalised language of his 'segregation reviews', the Mental Health Act documentation, and his psychiatry reviews. It was intended that he would be admitted for the 'treatment' of his 'challenging behaviour'. But, instead of the care, concern and understanding of family-style living, he is watched by 30 or as many as 50 interchangeable strangers who sit across his doorway in pairs, waiting to restrain him. I scoffed involuntarily when I heard that this was justified, in part because the bean bags on which he is forcibly restrained against his will must be referred to as 'safety pods'. It is just that kind of euphemism that allows the outrageous imprisonment of LeBron to continue without any serious challenge.

We shouldn't be in any doubt that this is primarily *a prison of ideas* – an ideology of "adaptive versus challenging behaviours". This ideology involves forgetting that those who cannot process their childhood maltreatment[10] will engage in survival behaviours when threatened, but still seek loving contact in between. The most painful thing about meeting him was the rebuffing of these attempts to connect and reciprocate. The unacknowledged hatred for him and the barely concealed wish to chastise and punish him was palpable, and yet unnameable. Everyone involved seemed to forget that their experiences with LeBron were changing their character as well. In her novel, the Mask of Apollo, author Mary Renault observed that "in hatred, as in love, we grow like the thing that we brood upon. What we loathe, we graft into our very soul".

10 LeBron was emotionally and physically abused as a child. He was neglected and often left in wet and dirty clothes. A family member was imprisoned, and there was domestic violence and family breakup. As an adult, he was assaulted by a member of his support staff, including severe bruising and finger marks where no lawful restraint would be used. None of these details were kept in mind by his hospital staff, most of whom were totally unaware of his history.

Chapter 9: Lucy and her parents

Blamed for loving too much

"If liberty means anything at all, it means the right to tell people what they do not want to hear".

George Orwell, *Politics and the English Language*, 1946

This chapter is about Lucy's foster parents and their relationship with Lucy. Alone with their own wisdom, they felt marginalised and blamed for wanting to remain in a parental role when she was an adult. We describe some aspects of our work with them and how we learned a lot from the process of supporting them.

Lucy was initially referred to our team by her social worker for help with apparent risks associated with secreting and hiding sharp items. She was due to be moved from a rather impersonal but modern and clean, locked-ward environment from which she had tried to escape several times. The social worker, charged with the task of "transition to adult services", implied that many 'crises' were occurring because Lucy's long-term foster parents, Sandra and Rob, could not 'cope' and were repeatedly calling the police when she would abscond.

We first attended professional's meetings, to which Lucy was not invited, to discuss these concerns. What was described was very chaotic; Lucy's birth family would be seen locally and she would insist on seeing them, or going drinking in public with people she had just met. Initially, it was strongly suggested that Lucy never refer to Sandra and Rob as her parents, especially now that she was an adult. It was strongly suggested that they were over-involved emotionally, headstrong in their advocacy for Lucy, and sometimes too restrictive of her freedom.

We noticed that the word 'crisis' seemed to be used a lot by everyone who talked about Lucy. It seemed that this referred to any time that Lucy wanted to do something that Sandra and Rob would, in her best interests, prevent her from doing. There was much alarm that this was a breach of

Lucy's rights and possibly even illegal. However, we were not convinced by the prevailing professional view of Sandra and Rob. Meetings would begin with too much praise of their years of commitment to Lucy, then progress to veiled criticism and then to the implication that they were incompetent, out of their depth, and lacking in reason.

Sandra called us one day to talk about Lucy. Contrary to the views passed on that she was over-involved and controlling, we found that she described offering freedoms to Lucy that were questionable, because Lucy seemed to be rather incapable of making the decisions in question. For example, she was allowed to restart contact with her birth parents and was later found inebriated on the street and brought home by her foster brother who was out looking for her. On discussing this with Sandra, she was surprised that we didn't automatically agree with the transitions team that Lucy living independently necessarily represented progress. Instead, we spoke of the lack of clarity about Lucy's level of functioning, and the apparent assumption that, when she put herself at risk, it was based on a full understanding of what she was doing. It seemed to us that Lucy was acting on impulse, not usually to manipulate others but to feel included in things, to be taken seriously – to exist as an important person in the minds of others.

Lucy responded worst when placed in group activities. The secreting of sharp items (which were always immediately handed over to Sandra and Rob when they asked) did not appear to have any immediate risk attached to it; instead, it seemed to function to create alarm about her. At the same time, we noticed the symbolism of sharp, penetrative items and their potential to harm – or defend oneself. We identified an inexplicable number of opportunities for Lucy to access such items and a lack of reviewed risks, almost as though she was set up to do it again and have another 'crisis'. Several members of her daycare team called her a 'collector' and saw the difficulty as laying within her condition, despite the apparent ease with which one-to-one support would preclude any such hoarding – both in terms of practically being able to do this, but also just not wanting to, because she didn't need to recruit attention. But such one-to-one support was seen as unaffordable, even infantilising.

This seemed to us to be a clue, a hint of something deeper in her memory. Yet even in immediate terms, it was clear that this would lead to people becoming more involved with Lucy, talking to her in concerned terms, wanting to know why she had done it, and this in and of itself seemed to reassure her – that she could become significant to others, even if only by being scary. It turned out that when she was with Sandra and Rob, such accumulations of objects were less likely, and they were much more likely if she was left at her day service or out and about and meant to occupy herself.

When actually interviewed by an advocate, Lucy stated that she would only be interested in moving to her own place when she was older, and only if she was next door to her parents. This illustrates that she had barely achieved object constancy[11], and was inappropriate for any kind of 'independent living' placement. This was taken to mean that it would require a long-term plan of a few months or years, but the spectre of sudden, unplanned moving was raised in response to any 'crisis' in professional meetings, almost to threaten Sandra and Rob and coerce them into giving up their identity as parental figures and instead become temporary carers with little emotional connection to Lucy.

We decided to offer an assessment using the Scale of Emotional Development – Short (Sappok *et al*, 2016). This assessment – an interview with key carers – essentially determines the level of emotional development that a person attains as described in Došen's stage model (see Chapter 2). Although this assessment determines the dominant stage attainment on a range of domains, in Lucy's case there was clear evidence that she was functioning almost exclusively in First Individuation (Stage 3), which is normally observed between 18 months and three years of age.

Whilst unwelcome, this finding had a very profound effect. Overnight, it altered the prevailing view held about Lucy in many important ways. Lucy could not decide whether she should be exposed to her birth family because she simply had no idea how to keep herself safe. She would be frightened, lonely and desperate if left to live in her own flat. She was not even suitable for the kinds of group activities she was expected to attend in day services. Suddenly, what was 'challenging behaviour' and 'crisis' was redefined as a developmentally appropriate behavioural response to neglect, and the only people who were determined that she should not be left to this neglect were Sandra and Rob.

11 The realisation that when a caregiver leaves the room, they still exist and will come back, usually happens about one year of age. This realisation can be undermined by neglect, where parents leave their babies for too long in the initial stages of development.

It is difficult to describe how such moments of change alter the powerful stories that are told about people with intellectual disabilities. Sandra said that, "All this time, it was like putting a square peg in a round hole. We knew it. We knew she needed us, that she will probably need us for years, or until we can't care anymore."

The assessment also led us to think very carefully about Lucy's history. Lucy was severely neglected as a baby and young child. Both parents were alcoholics and underfed her and her siblings. Food was occasionally left in bowls on the ground, in a locked room. While she was taken into the state system – one balks at calling it 'care' – at a very young age, Lucy was not offered anything stable until Sandra and Rob became her foster carers. She loved to be retold the story of the first time they met. Sandra and Rob needed a lot of resilience to get through the bureaucracy. They had to wait 'in a queue' – this was how they described it to Lucy – to wait until she would know that she would always be with them. Again, it is difficult to describe the deep meaning of the word 'always' when Sandra spoke of him. This 'always' element of Sandra and Rob's offer to the children and adults in their care was a direct challenge to the time-limited offer from the 'transitions' team. We noted that Sandra and Rob stopped talking about the proposed transition and began to talk to us in "forever" terms, for example, considering when they would have to retire as carers, and how to plan for Lucy to remain in their family home when they were no longer here.

When we complete an assessment of emotional development, we always offer a feedback session to everyone involved. In this session, we used the everyday expertise of everyone present to reference their children, grandchildren, nephews and nieces when considering if an action or comment by Lucy was *really* abnormal. In fact, it was clear that Lucy's freedom-seeking actions were entirely predicted by the First Individuation stage – to be taken seriously and involved. It was not really to obtain cigarettes or 'look normal' that she would abscond and ask strangers for "tabs". Conversely, hiding or not wanting to speak to others was not indicative of a sinister desire to hoard weapons or seriously harm herself; it was instead intended to seek safety when she felt abandoned in 'classroom' or 'work' settings. She was not ready for the expectation of functioning in peer groups.

We also noted that the narrative was changing. Instead of 'crisis', we encouraged the use of 'blip' or 'anxious episode'. In and of itself, this seems like just a change in word use, but it was in fact very powerful, representing the 'normalisation' of Lucy's actions as expected for her level of functioning. She sought to be recognised, taken seriously, included, but also struggled with some of the limitations that were very reasonable, like the need for personal care to be supervised in the community, to have one-to-one support in her day placement, and for a down time later for screen access. In addition, some limitation on the nature of some websites and internet content was required to protect her from sexual and financial exploitation. It was also understood that Lucy did not reason in logical terms and could be expected to struggle with the perspectives of others, without this seeming like a moral failure or a deliberate misunderstanding of the rules.

Sessions with Sandra and Rob, intended as advice for them, quickly became a two-way street. They shared experiences of caring for vulnerable young people with learning disabilities over many years. Crucially, they had grasped that activities and experiences that were appropriate for the person's chronological age, such as preparing complex meals, or using power tools, could be done by people with very limited emotional development. The key to balancing freedom with safety was finding the right level of involvement for each person. The children in their care who were very capable might only need them to be on the end of a phone. Others, though quite able in some ways, would barely leave their side, needing to know where they were at all times.

It's important to point out that both limited emotional development and significant adversity and trauma can have a similar effect; the need to be more intensely supported, supervised and comforted can address the need for safety either because safety was not available in the person's former life, or because they are simply not ready to strike out on their own. Sandra and Rob understood that they would have to be different for each individual child they cared for. Eventually, we noticed that we were no longer advising them; they were supporting us. This has remained something we are grateful for, up to and including their experiences enriching this book.

We could not believe more strongly that many people with learning disabilities, in the name of the principles of independence and choice-making – liberal political values – are expected to adjust to situations where they lack the love and support that they truly need. Over-estimation is endemic in the care system, reinforced by the financial need to reduce the burden on local authorities, as well as a service philosophy that comes from political principles, not a scientific understanding of emotional need. We often wonder how Sandra and Rob, despite years of messaging that they were ‘over-involved’, too ‘parental’, and ‘unprofessional’, resisted Lucy’s wider professional network without any external validation of their approach. Perhaps it is because they never lost sight of her need for love, and always remembered that any difficult situations were a product of her early experiences, that saw them through.

While the risk of being placed in an under-supported living situation faded away after our consultations, there are still concerns raised about Lucy from time to time at her college placement. This is usually because she is exposed to reminders of her life with the family of origin, which is both overly exciting, and frightening. Someone else might mention their family life, or a sibling, or say something insensitive about being adopted or fostered. Lucy may then ‘act out’ with Sandra and Rob, who sometimes seek support. However, the whole situation is much more calm because the family are not under threat of being broken up. Hence, Lucy is able to rely on Sandra and Rob to be there when she needs that safe haven.

Lucy remains in the care of Rob and Sandra. If she ever moves house, it will be to another family situation, when Sandra and Rob are too old. They will remain in close contact until finally separated by the grave.

We salute them.

Chapter 10: Helen

When will I be normal?

"The privilege of a lifetime is to become who you truly are".

Karl Jung

This chapter is an account of a counselling relationship between Victoria Shimmens and Helen. Helen was a young woman with mild intellectual disability, struggling with comparison to others, dependency on her family, and being culturally and religiously 'bound' into heterosexuality, which was incompatible with her authentic identity.

I had been seeing Helen for a year, for weekly counselling. Because of COVID this had to be online. In every session, the theme was really focused on 'normality'. She came with an agenda which seemed to imply being 'fixed', and she was referred for 'anxiety management' and low self-esteem.

Helen's Orthodox Jewish religion conflicted with feelings she had for other women. She had real trouble with the feelings of attraction and desire for several women, and I felt that this arose even with me as therapist in the transference. To pass anxiety to me, she would often talk about suicidal thoughts and plans at the end of the session, which would threaten the 'frame', i.e. make the session go beyond the agreed time.

Helen originally talked about a trusted person who had violated her sexually. She did not require prompting to talk about the event, which she described in a graphic and scripted manner, as though each time it was the first time the disclosure was being made. She would then guess at what my judgement was on this, and directly ask me to judge the meaning of this. I would try to redirect this to her own thoughts, but she would interrupt my response by saying, "I know, I know, I know, it's professional, we have different boundaries". Helen was asking for a friend's advice, rather than a counsellor's help with exploration.

Helen very much stayed in the 'victim' position (c.f. the Karpman drama triangle, described in more detail in Chapter 17). Partly, this seemed to reflect difficulty in admitting to feelings that would make her vulnerable to attack from her cultural beliefs (that it was immoral to be gay). This was very difficult to address, because it conflicted with my own moral values, which are for equality in sexual orientation. However, I had to respect her choice of values, and this led to a very careful approach of naming the dilemma she was in. If she was to adopt a gay identity, she said, "It would kill my family".

She told me that her family thought that she was "getting worse" because she was "talking about things". There was a strong feeling that the family needed to see the anxiety as an illness to be cured. I often used the analogy that counselling is not like having a broken bone fixed, and to feel better in the long run, upsetting thoughts would need to be felt.

Initially, Helen could not refer to "feeling gay" but, several sessions in, she said, "I have something big to tell you" and after a lot of approach-avoidance she said, "I feel gay – but I'm not". There were then sessions in which she would not raise this, almost to see if I would bring it up by asking about my recollections of previous sessions. In the sessions, I noticed that her feelings about the alleged assault were exciting, and that she thought about it in the shower, and dreamt about it. This did not fit completely with trauma, but did describe it as being "disgusting, I know it is", as though I had that judgement. Therefore, Helen's template was of someone disapproving of her sexuality. This was so internalised that she would screw up her features in apparent disgust, but there was a smirk as well. I had the uncanny feeling she could burst out laughing in the middle of this disgust.

Helen told us about a tutor she had who was in a lesbian relationship that was breaking up. She had strong feelings of attraction to this person. This was initially presented as a lifestyle that some part of her would like, but which could never be for cultural and religious reasons. Their relationship went beyond tutor and pupil, as the tutor would talk to her parents and accept hospitality from them, and there would be gifts exchanged at birthdays. The lessons kept being booked so that Helen could keep the relationship alive. Helen was very worried about this person's emotional state of mind (or perhaps what she imagined it to be) and knew all about her health and personal history. The tutor would openly talk to her professionals on the phone while Helen was there, which she then worried about. However, over time, the tutor appeared to tire of her.

The tutor's ex-partner had a son with autism, and the tutor suggested that the class he attended may be suitable for her, too. Helen was very angry about this, as it implied that she was not 'partner material', and it reinforced her status as a person with a learning disability who could not have relationships with people without disabilities. When the tutor ended the lessons, she was inconsolable in the following session.

Over time, I noted that Helen's lessons with the tutor were even used by the tutor to monitor her ex-partner. Helen had been sent on a personal errand of the tutor's which was in fact a cover story to see if she could catch sight of them. I encouraged Helen to think of the abusive element of this, which showed contempt for her. Helen often said that she felt angry, even vengeful, talking about reporting her tutor now that she knew they could never be together. There was little chance of her doing this. Instead, she got a new tutor whom she described initially as "professional", but then "too professional" (e.g., asking her not to use her phone in sessions). There was no personal sharing, which she did not like.

In formulating the case, I managed to state her wish to have a close relationship with a woman, which she did not disagree with. This was not specified as sexual. Throughout, I was aware that Helen was becoming strongly interested in me. She would playfully comment on her appearance, for example, her shirt, her hair, or make-up, which I would interpret, e.g., by saying, "Would you like me to like it?" While watching me for my reaction, she would respond by denying any such interest. This told me that Helen was afraid of her desires being named, because she perceived that the consequences would be catastrophic.

During our sessions, Helen's father died unexpectedly from an illness. At various different times, he had lived with her and lived away, which confused her. At times, he would call her 'special' but at other times she was angry that his absence affected the family. She started to see her older sister as the male head of the family. Her father was someone she could never contemplate talking to about the assault or her sexuality. When she did tell her mother and sister about her sexuality, fully expecting to be disowned, they were accepting of her feelings, but not the sexual identity.

Her response to his death was masked by her own illness which interrupted sessions. She was upset when I finally saw her, she cried and talked about missing him. At this time, I was just holding her emotions.

Sometimes she blamed herself, having had to nurse him for a time, but then she became ill herself and could not be around when he died. She didn't feel like she was a 'good enough daughter' and felt that she had missed the chance to see if he would accept her as she was, rather than being his 'princess'.

Helen continued to have difficulty with the question as to whether she would ever feel normal. It seemed that her project was to be adopted by a health professional rather than learning the skills to manage worries or overcome trauma. By continuing to ask, "What do you think I should do to feel better?" right up to the end, she was clinging to an idea of being changed to be accepted, rather than accepting herself for who she was. I wrote to her, talking about what therapy can change and what it cannot. In naming the limits of therapy, I had completed my therapy task, which was to help her formulate her psychological need, i.e., for a meaningful relationship with a woman, and that therapy could not offer this in the long term.

Everyone else seemed to imply that a further course of therapy would stop her feeling anxious – a false promise of normal, instead of affirming her personal value as she was. She was not bad, broken, or damaged. I stated that I accepted all of her. In my letter, I pointed out that she was a kind and loving person, and that we had shared a personal journey, and that this would always go on inside her. She talked of ending a chapter, so I mentioned that new chapters build on the story from previous chapters.

In our follow-up session, she confirmed that she had a new therapist and initially was saying she was "doing great". But as the session went on, she was still wanting me to tell her what was right, wrong, good or bad. She mentioned a new therapist who offered six structured sessions, but also said "she'll never be you". She kept saying how grateful and thankful she was. She said that "I would just have to get through to our session to survive a bad week". I felt some concern that no one was there for her like the therapy was. I referred to the letter and the internal dialogue with me. She said, "Yes, I ask myself what Victoria would say". She lamented the ending, and I reiterated that our therapy task had been completed – to name her dilemma, validate her experiences, to negate any message that she lacked human value.

In this, I hope that Helen in some ways understood that there is no normal. She did not know how to say what normal was. All the things she said that normal people do, such as 'not feeling like this', 'feeling happy', 'having jobs', having friends, being in a relationship, were all available to her and well within her grasp. But somehow, to fully achieve the feeling of being accepted, the significant others in her life would have to forsake the values of achievement, education and 'normality'. She had seen me accept her and had taken this with her, but she still faced contrary messages in many areas of her life. If she was to return for further work, we may look at strengthening the self-affirmation but would also consider how she can express who she truly is. While unconditional regard is a core feature of therapy and always part of sessions, I could not detect this in any of the other relationships in her life.

Reflecting further on the idea of 'normal', I started to feel some resentment at the meanings it carried for the people I was trying to help. It was quite a persecutory word, which implied not expressing a person's conflicted emotions. It stifled Hannah's ability to think through what she had experienced. I thought about 'normalising' treatments and attempts to help that were aimed at presenting with 'normal' behaviour, i.e., behaviour that other people would not consider embarrassing, confusing, annoying, or frightening. What, then, happens when a person has no way of expressing their need to be abnormal – because they need to process the fact that their life has not been normal, that it has been abusive and extreme? It cannot remain unexpressed, and therefore, when no one offers to listen properly, it becomes something else. It could become a voice that criticises a person; it could become low self-esteem; it could become soma (a physical symptom); it could lead us to say 'inappropriate' things; it could even become a non-shared experience, such as a hallucination. It cannot be accidental that almost all the people we see with any or all of these 'neuroses' and 'psychoses' seem to have been abused and/or neglected in some way or other.

And the need for the listener never leaves, until it is satisfied, and processing can begin. Confucius was thought to have said, "It cannot be when the root is neglected, that what springs from it will be well ordered." This seemed very apt to my experience of working with this kind, loving person with lots to give, who was forbidden from even knowing what was in her own mind.

Chapter 11: Murray

See me never

> *"I used to think the worst thing in life was to end up all alone. It's not. The worst thing in life is to end up with people who make you feel all alone."*
>
> Robin Williams

Murray is a 40-year-old man who was referred to our team for a behavioural 'treatment' for his 'aggressive' behaviours. Most of what we describe is an initial observation by Victoria Shimmens in his old day service where he never left the building, and then of a community trip to a local train museum, where he loved to look at the old steam engines, have a coffee and socialise. By the time of the observation, we had challenged the prevailing view that Murray was 'dangerous' or even psychopathic, which had been based on the fact that he enjoyed cartoons with lots of violence, like Tom and Jerry, and said that he wanted to do to his care team what happened to the characters. On assessing his emotional development it was clear that Murray could not yet separate fantasy and reality, but he did not actually enjoy seeing others in pain and was genuinely bonded to others.

Murray had not been ready for school and found his entire school career traumatic. He had been deeply unpopular with teaching staff, who called him "attention seeking" and – as we have seen in other cases – "manipulative". This carried on into adult residential placements. He had only very minimal contact with his family, less than once a year, yet he ached for their contact. He visibly grieved for the home manager, whom he referred to as "mam", when she moved on to another role. It was clear that his care team did not agree on the approach to Murray; some were convinced that he needed 'boundaries' (punishments) and others felt that he was treated disrespectfully by their colleagues. No one seemed to consider that his history of sexual abuse, inappropriate mechanical restraints, chronic neglect and virtual abandonment could have affected his ability to form relationships and function in a large group home.

My initial observation of Murray was at a day service where I was greeted by an agency member of staff. They were very focused on how dangerous Murray was and said that I would need guards on my arms to see him, because he nipped and bit. They started by telling me that he was having a 'terrible morning' and asked what we wanted to do. I said that we were just here to observe a typical day, but staff kept narrating about his difficult morning. I was with my community nurse colleague. The agency staff member was distracted by his phone; to start with, I was not aware that he was a member of staff, dressed as he was in a printed T-shirt and shorts. They talked about "behaviours" and "how many" there had been, but with no sense of understanding, compassionately, how he had come to act this way. They clearly saw it as based on rational choice, that they were in a battle of wills with someone whom they regarded as a threat and little else.

Murray was wearing dirty clothes and had food on his face. His clothes did not fit him, and he was underweight. He was in an old, derelict-looking building; the furniture was moved around, and much of it was under-used. Where he spent his time was dull, lacking in stimulation. It was as if the building itself was hopeless, hapless, aimless.

Murray came down to the locked door and said, "What's your name? Why you here?" Murray always talked in three-word phrases and would repeat the question until answered. He asked, "You with me?" I told him my name and where we were from – "Come to meet you". He was happy about this. The day care worker said, "He'll act up for you; he likes to have an audience". There was a staff member who seemed to be 'chasing' him with a pair of shoes to "go to the activities room". He was avoiding putting the shoes on. He hid behind the corner and jumped out, saying, "Pretend, pretend, pretend". They would then ask if he wanted to go to the 'games' room and he would say yes, but then he would refuse to put his shoes on. He would jump out on them, saying, "Get a fright, get a fright". It was clearly a game, but I could feel them becoming annoyed with him. Eventually, he put his shoes on when he was ready, and he went over to the activities centre.

What followed was a whole one-man show of 'The Wizard of Oz'. He had not yet formed a strong sexual identity, being mainly at the Socialisation stage (see Chapter 2) with only some aspects of First Individuation, so he did not mind playing male or female characters. Some people in his care team would engage with this pretend play, while others would not at all, leaving him somewhat confused. Murray often said, "Me not like you" when others would not engage in his games. This was usually with people who expected him to behave in a 'classroom' fashion, sitting quietly doing formal learning, or at least not being a challenge. But Murray's development had not reached this level.

Things stared to escalate when he was doing his 'performance'. There were some instruments in the room, but these would not work properly. Instead of distracting him with interesting activities, they tried to tell him why it would not work. He instead tried to get to instruments in the next room. The staff could not allow this, and eventually, because of risk, they wanted to take him out of the environment, for which he would have to put his shoes on again. This led to Murray throwing one of the shoes at a staff member. The staff member said, "Okay, everyone out, everyone out" and in the chaotic melee that followed, he was eventually led out in a walking two-person restraint either side. Murray was both excited and animated, but also visibly anxious during this whole episode.

Everyone working with Murray seemed stressed, irritated by him, burnt out, and over-focused on his compliance. There was no fondness, no warmth. They did not see his fun side; they did not delight in his games or his interests; they simply saw him as a management problem. We noted their relief at the idea of him being moved on, and no longer being responsible for him. They did not want the bond to remain, or for us to successfully maintain their bond; they had lost any love for him, if it was ever there.

It seems that this was always the case with Murray – that the over-estimation of his emotional development caused others to believe that enjoying, engaging, and tolerating his games and play was somehow more than he deserved; that he should behave well, sit down, get on with formal learning, and stop being emotionally demanding. As a result, the team he was working with, and perhaps his family of origin, wanted him to go, to be someone else's responsibility.

Our intervention was not really very complex. We pointed out that he had the emotional needs that are usually seen before the third birthday, that this would require intensive, parental-style support; we told his professionals to stop worrying about learning independence skills, and to think more about forming a permanent bond with him; that there would always be a 'battle of wills' from a person who simply wanted to feel that others who were with him were listening, that he could have an effect on them and feel that his wishes were taken seriously, and that when he was thwarted and lashed out, that they would not withdraw from him, hurt him, or want rid of him. What was most distressing about Murray's case was the occasional phone calls from his father, whom he would desperately ask to see. His father would promise to come 'soon', but never appeared. It seemed the loving mirror we all need from others was reflecting a false promise, and we wondered if anyone really loved him at all. Did anyone want to see him, or was all of his human contact begrudged, hiding a wish for him to be gone? Many of Murray's games could, therefore, be seen as rather desperate attempts to engage, and his questions about who was 'with' him an anxious preoccupation about whether he was going to be abandoned.

The observation ended with us being ushered into a staff office so that one of the senior workers could assure us that he was dangerous, aggressive, manipulative and incredibly hard to work with. They wanted to make the case that he did not belong there. We already knew this, but for reasons that would have shocked them to hear. Of his more egregious sins, the worst one seemed to be "stealing staff's food and drink". It did not need much psychoanalysing to link this to the emotional 'depletion' that the staff felt in Murray's presence. There was so much horror of him; he could clearly see this on their faces.

I left feeling that the poverty in Murray's environment was not just about the redundant furniture, the old building he was often left in, and the lack of any fun activities that would hold his attention. The staff were well trained in behavioural work, 'safe' restraint[12], and risk assessments. But they had no fondness for him; they didn't want him, because they felt he was too demanding, too oppositional, and asked too much of them emotionally.

This illustrates again one of the key points of this book: that an accurate assessment of the emotional development of people who are described in terms of their 'challenging behaviour' is essential when providing them with care. Murray functioned at the Socialisation Stage, and therefore, as we have seen in Chapter 2, he was very focused on emotional safety and whether he was valued or rejected as a person. To explore the world, Socialisation requires a strong attachment bond with someone who adores

12 We mean "safe" in the sense that he was unlikely to be physically injured when his restraints were applied according to the staff physical restraint training. We do not imply that it was not traumatic for Murray to be forced to the floor, dominated by the physicality of the staff, and humiliated.

one. While some emotional expression is possible, there is no empathy for others and so the person may seem sadistic or cruel. If the person is overestimated in emotional development, this will be judged morally and invite negative consequences so that the person will 'learn'. In fact, negative and aversive responses will cause the person to become more desperate in their actions. While caregivers should expect to feel guilt at their emotional responses to the person's aggressiveness or other behaviours that concern them, their constancy and unwavering support tend to win out, strengthening and deepening the bond so that eventually there is no risk of them being asked to leave.

Murray had not reached this point in his development, and it was difficult to locate anyone in his life who was committed in the long term. Everyone in his environment wanted him to leave and not see them anymore. This could not be expressed directly but was instead acted out through multiple referrals to the community team to deal with his behaviours. Despite our intervention, the idea that Murray consciously and deliberately attacked his care staff to gain 'control at their expense' remained powerful and eventually led to his being rejected from the service.

An update on Murray

Murray moved to a new home which was much more focused on the relationship with him. Despite a rocky start and a focus on 'behavioural incidents', reports from these incidents mentioned how sorry they felt for Murray when he was anxious or upset, and illustrated thinking that reflected their attempt to understand what he was experiencing. They were equally concerned about the disappointment Murray felt by his family's promises and would even compare him to their own family members. This team took over his day care responsibilities and took him into the community with an appropriate balance of risk assessment and, bearing in mind his wish to socialise, determined that he would become known and liked by the local café staff and its clientele.

Murray continued to present some difficulties for his care team – for example, if he saw a fire engine, he would be convinced that there was a fire at home, and would become extremely, inconsolably distressed, and on one occasion he needed to be escorted home by the police. Yet this was not a threat to the placement, or a precursor to hospitalisation through the language of 'crisis' or 'mental health breakdown'. It was instead understood as a sign of earlier trauma, which his new care team were determined to overcome via their loving relationship with him. He continues to live at this home with many happy times and where he feels wanted, supported to explore, and comforted. In short, he has found a family, and found a place where people love him and would miss him if he was gone.

Chapter 12: Sonny

The absolute minimum

"Fantasy is hardly an escape from reality.
It's a way of understanding it."

Lloyd Alexander

This chapter describes details and some reflections of the first meeting between Victoria Shimmens and Sonny, a young man with an intellectual disability sent to the team because of concerns about 'psychosis' related to epilepsy, which had been ruled out by his neurologist and his psychiatrist. Although he was receiving medication to 'calm' him, his team did not believe that this was sufficient, and were shocked when the psychiatrist referred him to psychology. Reluctantly, they agreed to meet the psychology team and have a formal assessment of emotional development.

Initially, on receiving this referral, I contacted the care team to receive the incident forms. The incident forms described "nasty comments" from Sonny to the staff, which they felt were completely unacceptable. Typically, Sonny did not really want to engage with his team to do activities with them. Having moved out of his family home recently, he struggled to adjust. He stayed in touch with his family on FaceTime, but this only caused him to feel excluded when he saw other family members being included. When prompted to go out or engage in daily activities of living, Sonny sometimes refused and would say that he did not like the people allocated to work with him. He made unrealistic, fantastical threats such as putting staff in a castle, locking them up in a prison, or having dogs set upon them which would eat them.

I visited Sonny at home. He was a little wary when I was first shown in, and was prompted by staff to "Tell Victoria about where we went yesterday" or "What did you do on Thursday?" His carer, Cilla, then said, "I am going to work in the office, and you can talk to Victoria about anything you want". This seemed to move swiftly from strong prompting and authority to asking Sonny to suddenly account for himself without support. There was something a little dismissive or avoidant about this

– it came across that the staff team had nothing to learn, and I should give Sonny 'treatment' to make him behave better or even simply obey instructions. They would say, "He doesn't listen to us", but this really meant "He does not obey, and can become angry". Implicitly, I felt I was being asked to make him comply and stop being angry.

Sonny told me about dreams he was having. One was about flying in a free and exhilarating way, another was about being magical and powerful, and yet another was about being able to go wherever he wanted. He remembered his dreams vividly. I thought about how dreams can carry with them a wish, just below consciousness, and it made me think about Sonny's desires and wishes. He seemed to be constricted by his environment, where no one wanted to talk about such things. He was just expected to behave well; to be a 'good boy' as described in Freud's latency period, where children are compliant, studious, and relatively easy to care for.

I noticed that Sonny had not reached this level, emotionally; sometimes he did not understand completely where imagination ended, and reality began. We were not surprised by this, but his care team struggled to accept it. Talking about his dreams as though they were real was seen as over-excitement, dangerous, "epileptic" and, if not discouraged, they felt it could become "psychotic". Strangely, they both encouraged him to depict his dreams by drawing pictures, but also disapproved of any expressions to do with his imaginings. He began to tell me about memories of his nephew, and thoughts about comments from his mum that were intended to be humorous but were clearly experienced as hurtful and rejecting by Sonny.

Sonny had a longstanding relationship with Cilla, the team manager. A prior arrangement of care involved Cilla spending time at the family home, before he moved to his current home. Clearly, Sonny did not consent to moving out, but it was done in his "Best Interest", a strange legal term in which professionals can make decisions for others if they are deemed to "lack mental capacity" to make life decisions. The explanations on file were about adult independence and freedom, but in fact, Sonny had little freedom. While he continued to be in the presence of disapproving others, there was less in the way of a mix of love and disapproval – it was nearly all disapproval.

Sonny started to tell me about a memory of his nephew and brother. Something had happened where he was physically hurt during a disagreement. He started to feel angry, and said, "That's not nice, is it?"

This incident was, as he remembered it, that his nephew had knocked an ornament over and hurt himself, but Sonny got the blame and was deeply emotionally hurt by this. However, despite the intention to deflect blame onto Sonny, he had a strong streak of resistance to taking the blame for this event. Sonny was considered to have a 'delusional' belief that he had a magic marble which could somehow take revenge on people who admonished him. He often spoke to the marble, confidently expecting its magic to smite others on his behalf. In one sense, this was a delusion; the marble was incapable of harming anyone, and indeed Sonny didn't seem to register that the marble hadn't actually hurt anyone. However, it is common for young children and some adults with ID to believe that magic exists in reality, and indeed this lingers on in adult suspension of belief. Indeed, it might be argued that we need to have this capacity in order to have creative imagination. If we could not imagine the impossible, how could we invent fairy tales, suspend belief while watching fictional films, or even have any creativity? It struck me that he was trying to use his marble-talk to resist the collapse of his self-esteem. This might tell us something about so-called 'delusions' in people who have no conventional way of expressing their feelings of abandonment and rejection, either through the terrible pain of remembering their past treatment, or because they don't have the cognitive capacity to do this.

I was reminded of many other cases where a person who did not understand the feelings and needs of others was being judged on moral grounds when they did not have the emotional skills to be this wily or manipulative. In fact, the words 'nasty', 'attention seeking', 'manipulative', 'unacceptable', 'horrible' and other personal judgements were frequently used in these cases' care plans.

As the visit progressed, I spent some time validating his feelings about his memories, saying that I could see how it was hard for him. It seemed important to properly listen to Sonny and open up otherwise shut down conversations. By saying, "I am sure that wasn't so" or, "I am sure she did it for good reasons", or "let's not think about that, let's think about nice things", his care team *consciously* wanted to help Sonny to feel OK, but this actually stopped Sonny from processing his losses and hurt feelings.

So, when Sonny talked to his magic marble, this allowed him some imaginary revenge on those whom he felt to be rejecting him. He would say things he wanted to come true, like having a girlfriend, making a staff member his girlfriend, and hurting people who had thwarted him. This is where he would ask the marble to put people in a dungeon or in a river, etc. It is important to say that he never acted on any of those fantasies. His staff team felt that this should be stopped, and the family had asked for it to be thrown away, so, clearly, they did not see how this was Sonny's attempt to deal with frustration and sorrow. They called it "bizarre behaviour" and "inappropriate" and "not nice to do". However, it struck me as something that allowed him to explore, in a limited way, feelings that are hard to keep inside.

We had already completed a standardised assessment of emotional development, which had suggested that Sonny was functioning, emotionally, at about 1½ to three-year level, but several members of the care team had left or joined, and Cilla had forgotten to share the training session and our Emotional Development Workbook. Cilla disapproved of what she called "people having a soft approach", by which she meant that Sonny should be told in no uncertain terms what was right and what was wrong, although punishments were not formally used. I suspected that, if Sonny was seen as having been 'in a funny mood' or 'nasty', community activities would be cancelled. Some favoured activities were made unavailable, such as visits to coffee shops, because of an 'incident' in which he had said something socially gauche to a member of the public. I felt that this was an overreaction, designed to teach him a lesson.

Cilla showed me some 'care plans' that involved the unwarranted use of medication to calm him in response to his mood. Much of his care plan was about staff "not reacting" to him, which is very hard to do and actually came across as sulking, so these care plans were intended to punish him and discourage his expression of negative feelings. Some of it was totally inappropriate and breached guidelines on safe and appropriate care, leading to a formal safeguarding process.

There was also an element of potential envious 'spoiling'[13]. Cilla seemed to struggle with our ideas, which contradicted her strongly held belief that the care team should "give him the bare minimum of attention". We promoted connection and help for Sonny to process his emotions. She told me that "a member of our staff has done some psychology and is going to write a behaviour plan", but I pointed out that this would need to be in collaboration with our community team because it was not best practice. Not only should care teams not mark their own homework, but it was very clear to us that Sonny needed an attachment-based intervention and not behavioural guidelines, especially guidelines which we suspected may have turned into subtle (and not-so-subtle) forms of maltreatment. Cilla would chip in to comment that she had "worked with the family for years", would "come in on days off", and would be called if Sonny said "something nasty" to his team.

It felt as though Sonny was getting a lot out of my proximity and my interest in exploring his thoughts and feelings. Conversations with staff always kept being moved on to the next task or subject, and they steered away from negative emotions. They would advise people to keep clear of subjects that were conflicted in him, as this could "cause a seizure". However, I felt that this was a defence against their own fears that Sonny would present his anxiety, which they did not want or feel able to process.

Despite the distracting interloping from the care team, I remained very interested in Sonny's imagination and his potential for affectionate bonding, so we kept talking for the hour of my visit. Inevitably, however, I had to leave for another appointment. At this moment, I felt as though I did not want to leave Sonny, because it felt like I was leaving him to be with people who did not care about him. While there were people present, they were either

13 The psychoanalyst Melanie Klein proposed, disconcertingly, that a basic feature of human emotional life and our resulting personality is based on envy. Someone else always has something that we covet; the child envies the power and control of the adult, young adults covet the assets of the old; the old covet the youth of the young; the poor envy the rich; the unloved envy the loved, and so on. Envy, unlike conscious jealousy, is paranoid, and linked to destroying, attacking and denigrating. When envy dominates, the envious person does not just wish to have what they covet. They would rather destroy anything good or worthwhile so that everyone has nothing. Klein's idea helps explain why some people can suddenly and irrationally attack others, seemingly unfairly or in a random way. In the envious state of mind, a person feels that others are against them, including authority figures, or even the world. The counterpoint to envy is appreciation, gratitude and empathy. These qualities are developed during secure Attachment relationships, so that our envy eventually stops dominating. However, for some, envy remains strong so that they continue to struggle with others having something that they do not and will try to spoil good relationships between other people and devalue what they say or offer. This shores up their self-esteem, which can be very fragile, but also leads to serious problems in relating to others since the personality remains fundamentally immature. To learn more about Klein, visit melanie-klein-trust.org.uk

working on laptops, working in the office, or otherwise turned away. I was being avoided and there was a pointed lack of interest in what I was saying. This was acknowledged by comments such as, "He is okay while you're here, we had a right morning though" and, "He'll probably kick off later".

As I got up to leave, Sonny got up and walked me to the door. His carer told him to say goodbye. I said, "If it's all right with you, I would like to come and see you again. I'm really interested in what you have to say." He said, "Yes, please". As I left the building, I was not convinced that his care team really wanted me to visit again. I could hear comments over my shoulder containing accusations of 'ignoring' certain staff members, like he owed *them* all equal attention, when any and all of the care team felt they had permission to ignore him for the whole of their shift.

It's important to say very clearly that the staff were not impolite or *consciously* unkind to Sonny. There was, however, a powerful ongoing dynamic with Cilla and her care team. In supervision, I reflected with my supervisor on a feeling of hopelessness that they could ever feel deep affection for Sonny; that underneath, there was deep anger at and contempt for him. This was, I felt, a direct consequence of his anxiety at being pushed out by his family combined with a profound lack of any thinking about his deep emotional pain. He was forced to act out his anger because no one would help him turn it into words. In his work with forensic clients, Professor Brett Kahr (2021) has called this the difference between insults and spears. Words can hurt, but this is always preferable to being physically attacked. Therefore, we should talk to people about their emotional pain, and not discourage this for fear that they might become upset.

If we do not risk insults, we will risk spears.

Sonny's team could not see that refusing to talk to him about his frustration was denying him human connection. I did not find it very difficult to talk with him, and he could almost immediately explain his feelings and benefit from doing so. I will not forget the warmth and expectation in his "Yes, please". I did see him again for several such visits, and although the frequent use of medication to sedate him went down, Cilla continued to take him to the psychiatrist and report incidents of 'seizures' as justification for continued and even increased use of strong psychotropic medications. What he really needed, and will continue to need, was true empathic listening by someone he liked and trusted. What he got was physically adequate care coupled with emotional coldness and, sometimes, open hostility when he was anxious or upset. This was overlaid with a medical story about 'seizures' requiring 'medication' to make him 'well', a totally incompatible narrative to the conversation we were trying to have with him.

When I left my role some months later, this kind of secure attachment was still missing for him. I made sure that I told my team it was an unmet need, and I still wonder if there is anyone in Sonny's life with any real interest in him. As for my attempt to connect, though it felt real and I knew that my colleagues would keep trying to make it and take on board the work I had done with him, it seemed to remain vulnerable to being rubbished, and any benefit denied. Behind the increased insistence of routinely presenting Sonny's case as a medical case of psychotic obsession with his marble, causing epileptic 'seizures', causing aggression, which required medication and some form of unspecified disapproval (which turned into sulking), was an envious resentment at being offered something helpful: a way to understand his limited emotional development, and then talk to him about what was making him feel sad and abandoned.

However, I knew that his potential remains. In 1937, psychoanalyst Melanie Klein said, "Feelings of love and gratitude arise directly and spontaneously in the baby in response to the love and care of his mother." Since he was offered only the bare minimum, Sonny had only the minimum of love and gratitude to his care team, but I was hopeful that one day, when others had taken a more genuine interest in his emotional life, he could reciprocate and there would be a happier life available to him.

References

Kahr B (2021) Insults and Spears: tribulations of forensic disability psychotherapy. In Frankish P, Beail N & Skelly A (eds) *Trauma and Intellectual Disability: Acknowledgement, Identification and Intervention*. West Sussex: Pavilion Publishing.

Klein M (1937) cited in Mann D (2013) *Love and Hate: Psychoanalytic Perspectives*, p.79. London: Routledge.

Chapter 13: Jeremiah

Let's have meetings to avoid him

"It's not Denial. I'm just selective about the reality I accept."

Bill Watterson

This chapter describes the experience of attending many meetings about Jeremiah, a young man considered complex and with profound and multiple disabilities. Despite many past failures of care, the many professionals involved desperately wanted to help him, and this led to regular weekly multidisciplinary meetings (MDTs), which were consciously intended to lead to a well-led, effective and co-ordinated set of interventions.

Allan Skelly felt it was necessary to describe something of this process to explain how such meetings are not straightforward and tend to avoid painful awareness of the things that cannot be magically changed, while actually causing the relationships around the person to be temporary and unstable. There were several, seemingly incompatible stories about the person, which we try to draw out. These stories are laden with great power and are supposed to be of great help to people, but we find them limited and constraining, and in urgent need of critique, if not consignment to history.

Jeremiah was referred to the community learning disabilities team by his school as he approached his 18th birthday. The referral contained a lot of concerning information; he was described as unmanageable and regularly violent, often unable to attend school due to violence towards taxi drivers and his carers. At school, he was reported to be learning very little, despite the school being commissioned to work with the most challenging cases.

Local services regularly held 'transitions meetings', which are intended to identify young people with ongoing complex needs who may need to carry on seeing specialist services when they become adults. Previous experience of this process was frustrating, mainly because children's services would identify work for our team that they had been unable to do, or which was incomplete because the children's services were unable to offer more than short-term work, or because the person had been on the waiting list for so long they had simply passed their 18th birthday. Usually, one model of care (e.g., medication for a chemical imbalance, behavioural interventions to 'discourage' so-called 'challenging behaviours', sensory interventions to address a 'narrow zone of tolerance') was dominant and no room was allowed for new ways of thinking[14].

Prior to any formal referral, I was invited to attend an Education and Health Care Plan (or EHCP) meeting without the time to gather any context or pre-assessment information. It is easy to expect that we would do this, but in practice, we are often invited to these meetings with only one or two days' notice and have full diaries in between. Sometimes we attend with almost no knowledge of the person, though many people in the meetings expect us to already know the case well, to have automatically accepted the person for intervention, and await us to announce our fully formed care plan, as though it has some hitherto unknown miracle ingredient. This can occur without a realistic grace period in order to get to know the person.

Attendees of such meetings may be familiar with how procedural they are. Many aspects of the person's life are described, with multiple sections requiring many details to be filled out. One might expect that a single professional would lead on this, and indeed our own organisation intends for one person to be the 'care co-ordinator'. However, this role is often pushed onto others, because the bureaucracy involved is a significant strain on the named person. It didn't help that individual professionals were able to easily transfer the role to someone else on the electronic system, and then formally end their involvement. Jeremiah was no exception in this regard; the meeting organiser's first action in the ECHP meeting was to say; "I have only attended two of these meetings, I have been unable to contact the parents, and I will be discharging the case next week, prior to my secondment to another service". He then asked me if I would be leading the case, as "His primary needs are behavioural".

Such events are not rare in our experience, but they never cease to feel like being pushed into a river just at the top of a waterfall and being expected to steer everybody else to safety immediately. The 'waterfall' is, of course, the imminent collapse of the family or the care agency. While it seems that everyone who attends is keen to limit their own

14 Typically, in the medical model, a person diagnosed with ADHD, mood 'disorder', or autism spectrum disorder would simply be placed upon stimulant or major tranquilising medication – powerful drugs intended to (but lacking strong evidence for their ability to) address behavioural issues or mood. These children almost always had multiple childhood adversities with serious concerns reflected in formal safeguarding procedures, but this had not been addressed by psychological or psychotherapeutic means.

responsibility and to look for others to offer actual work that might help the person, there is also a great imperative for someone to relieve the anxiety of the hastily formed group.

Jeremiah was defined according to powerful, constraining stories. These stories, including our preferred way of explaining his case (Narrative 4: The trauma & attachment-informed approach), are constructed in professional language, which represents reality but is not reality. Since human thoughts cannot grasp all physical reality, the ideas that explain a person's situation are always lacking.

However, we believe that some are more lacking in validity – and therefore usefulness to people like Jeremiah – than others.

1. Jeremiah framed as a man with medical conditions (suffers – victim)
2. Jeremiah framed as a man who is discriminated against and needs to be empowered (rescued)
3. Jeremiah framed in terms of his behaviour (persecutor)
4. Jeremiah considered from a trauma- and attachment-informed perspective (none of the above).

Narrative 1: Jeremiah has a mental disorder (prior to referral and meetings 1–2)

The outgoing 'care co-ordinator' did attempt to tell us about Jeremiah prior to backing out of the case. It was first stated by way of an introduction to the case that "Jeremiah has ADHD, learning disability, depression, and an anxiety disorder". The most successful contact with Jeremiah was his three-monthly clinic appointments with a child psychiatrist. The psychiatrist's letters to the general practitioner had a set template: (1) diagnosis list; (2) medication list; (3) medication changes; (4) a paragraph about what Jeremiah's care worker had found difficult since the last clinic appointment, such as "outbursts when he doesn't get his own way", "getting himself stressed when asked to go home", and "agitated episodes"; and (5) plan, usually an increase in a medication designed to treat low mood in the general population.

These letters never attempted to trace his actions to his past experiences, only to the perceived benefit or harm from the latest medication change. It is striking that the main source of information in most cases of such letters is the opinion of the carer, and sometimes a comment or two from the person themselves, if they are verbal. It is very unlikely that the person or their carer will be aware of the debates and controversies surrounding the use of strong mind-altering drugs, such as placebo effects, suppressed negative outcome studies, or drug withdrawal effects in control groups.. (The issues with the long-term use of powerful drugs affecting the nervous system for the purpose of reducing distress, or making a person's behaviour more socially acceptable, is explored in much more depth in the case of Jennifer, in Chapter 16.)

In the medical model as applied to Jeremiah's case, he is seen as a victim, or *sufferer*, of a medical ailment. This ailment is not his personal responsibility, and it is strongly implied that his anxiety, distractibility, angry feelings and actions etc. are imposed by the condition. This has the positive effect of preventing moral judgement on Jeremiah when he has hurt someone else, damaged property, or hurt himself.

Narrative 2: Jeremiah is oppressed and should strive for independence and liberty (meetings 2–3)

This idea of Jeremiah was presented in multi-agency meetings by his social worker, in alliance with a professional advocate. To some extent, his family also agreed that his main problem was that he could not access the services that could help him throughout his life. There was certainly something to be said for this view in terms of the simple evidence on file – despite over 30 meetings being held over the five years from the age of 13 to 18 years, only three actual assessments were carried out: a psychiatric assessment at the age of 14 leading to his medication prescription; an 'opt in' meeting at the age of 15, which is an initial triage assessment, which led to no further intervention as the professionals and family argued about missed appointments; and an assessment at the age of 17 by a psychologist which was listed as a 'consultation', but concluded that his behaviours were "not appropriate for our team". This latter conclusion was confusing because clearly Jeremiah was extremely distressed at times and his behaviour demonstrated his often-extreme feelings.

We noted that the people who took this position might be considered 'rescuers' within the drama triangle[15] which we explore in full later. Within this 'rescuer' role, which is comfortable in the short term but unsatisfactory in the longer term, the professional may attempt to identify the person as a 'victim' of a 'persecutor'. In this instance, it was strongly implied that by failing to 'treat' Jeremiah with medical, psychological, and occupational interventions, the healthcare professionals were persecuting him. Their intervention – advocacy – was therefore intended to identify this 'injustice' in the form of failure to access effective treatments. Privately, we hypothesised that they were in fact (unconsciously) discharging their own anxiety about Jeremiah's perceived lack of progress by attacking the health professionals as incompetent and avoidant. We perceived a mix of justifiably standing up against the failure to really help Jeremiah to process his trauma, and a wish for someone to take on his care, so they would not have to worry about it anymore. This was rather vengeful and un-empathic, with the implication that they might take up formal complaints against the children's service. What was evoked in reality, however, was a series of rational responses about the processes involved that diverted blame (and therefore shame) from the healthcare system.

In turn, the health professionals explained that the family had missed several appointments; they were currently facing a huge demand and could not prioritise a person if they did not show up for their assessments; individual practitioners had 'valid' reasons for not carrying on working with Jeremiah, such as leaving their posts, being on sick leave for extended periods, waiting for other people to do assessments prior to their own, other teams (such as the crisis team) taking over, etc. Each individual instance of approach-avoidance by the professionals had a plausible explanation for not helping Jeremiah to *sit down and talk* about what was upsetting him, and yet, stepping back, there had been many years where everything seemed to conspire to prevent any real connection.

Our organisation was not our enemy; for many years it was supportive of our work and allowed us to practice without micromanaging. However, we 'diagnosed' organisational systems that prevented connection to emotionally painful information when dealing with the people of the area who needed its help. We think, following Bion (1961) and Stokes (1994),

15 Described in more detail in Chapter 17, the Karpman drama triangles include a 'triangle of conflict' which includes three interchangeable 'positions' in interpersonal relationships where there is conflict, namely, victim, rescuer, and persecutor.

that organisations lack collective consciousness of how their systems become avoidant and defensive, and thus, when scandals are exposed, they engage in ineffective 'learning' which tends to scapegoat, divert and deny, and thus fail to prevent future scandals (Skelly *et al*, 2022).

Examples of the organisation engaging in such unthinking and unhelpful processes in Jeremiah's case included the strong tendency to hold weekly meetings and argue about attendance at these, instead of focusing on meeting Jeremiah and engaging in a conversation with him. The family did experience painful emotions about his perceived behavioural problems, so did not always take up the appointments offered, partly because of fear of being judged negatively, and partly because the value of what was being offered was not explained to them. The organisation's policy of "two strikes and you are out" when people Do Not Attend (DNA) was communicated by a set form of letter, which simply stated that the person or family had failed to attend "and therefore your case will be discharged from our service". While the letter involved an invitation to be re-referred via the general practitioner, in reality, this would place the person at the bottom of a waiting list, which could be relatively short (up to several months or even years).

Even when accepted and appointments offered and attended, Jeremiah's family could experience assessments that were not very focused (such as a general health assessment) largely due to the healthcare trust having policies about collecting certain information, such as levels of alcohol use, employment and accommodation status, etc. This could seem tone-deaf to Jeremiah's concerns and come across as more about the organisation's needs. A 'care co-ordinator' would be assigned as a matter of policy, but as we have seen above, they were often ambivalent, if not resentful of being assigned by an impersonal process without discussion, leading to the impulse to pass this role on to others. They often simply referred to another team instead on flimsy grounds. The multidisciplinary discussions and meetings that would follow could be characterised as arguments about the case "not being my job".

The frustration with these organisational defences and the inability of the system to become aware of what it was doing, was reflected in the viewpoint of the advocate and social worker, that Jeremiah was essentially being denied the healthcare treatment to which he was entitled. Not being clinicians, they looked on at repeated attempts at poorly focused assessments and saw an organisation that was simply not doing its job. Rationalisations within the meetings took up much of the discussion but failed to resolve this in any way – everyone in the meeting felt that someone else was failing in their role, never themselves, and never as a group.

Our own view was that this narrative had rightly identified that Jeremiah needed something different, but it wrongly assumed that this was about his right to healthcare being denied because healthcare professionals were prejudiced against disabled people, or just being bad at their jobs. In Karpman's drama triangle, 'rescuing' always fails, because it lacks empathy and places others in the 'persecutor' or the 'victim' positions, which only evokes defensive responses and fails to help with real, creative actions that might give a new understanding of a person's predicament.

Narrative 3: Jeremiah's 'challenging behaviour' needs to be managed (meetings 3–12)

To the extent that Jeremiah's life experiences were discussed, this took the form of describing him by the actions he took that others found exasperating, which was often paraphrased as "he had a behaviour"[16]. These included running into shops and hiding in staff only areas, going into Emergency Care departments with small overdoses of four to six paracetamol, ringing his social worker in the middle of the night, throwing his TV remote at his mother or sister, and generally behaving in ways that brought focus to him and evoked extreme annoyance. When we asked about life experiences and how these acts might signal more than just 'attention seeking', and might be symbolic of a deeper, desperate need for something to be recognised, we were politely moved on, as though this wasn't appropriate business for an organisation that helps people with their distress.

Let's consider for a moment what 'attention seeking' can mean. In and of itself, it is neutral. However, it is rarely used in a neutral way. It tends to mean 'annoyingly distracting', 'deliberately emotionally dependent' (rather than having limited emotional development), 'selfish', and/or some other meaning that implies a *moral failing*, rather than a physical or emotional need.

16 Positive Behaviour Support (PBS) advocates are at pains to point out that using 'behaviour' only to refer to 'challenging behaviour' is not correct, and that most of our actions are either neutral (not functioning to meet our needs) or adaptive (meeting our needs). In practice, we find that behavioural approaches are incredibly focused on challenging behaviours and how to prevent or address them. While this is understandable, it comes to define the person as essentially a 'challenging person', which was never the aim of PBS.

The idea of 'behaviour management' grew from the work of behavioural psychologists who broadly followed the ideas of BF Skinner, via a system of reward (positive reinforcement), escape from an aversive consequence (negative reinforcement), or via negative or unwanted consequences to actions (punishment). However, including the word 'management' can be attributed to the educationalist Lee Canter who, in the 1970s, used Skinner's principles to design a system which would prevent individual pupils in schools from disrupting a whole class. Note that this was to help the teacher and the group of learners, not the individual. This is important to realise – that when groups of professionals or carers talk about 'managing behaviour' they are usually talking about what *they* need. Now, PBS explicitly states that its purpose is to meet the needs of the individual, but in reality, loose and fuzzy language, about 'strategies', 'support' and 'dealing with' behaviour, confuses this principle, often until progress becomes seen as the person being quiescent and not presenting difficulties for those around them.

Furthermore, a strong wish from professionals and carers to achieve compliance in the person can militate against any conversation that questions their own responses and potential influence on the person's well-being. No one likes feeling that they are to blame for a difficulty caused to others. Yet, when 'managing behaviour', the very idea of doing so implies that up until now it has not been done properly. We have already met a challenge to the fantasy that all behaviour can, with appropriate behaviour guidance, be made non-challenging to other people by considering emotional development and how this can be limited by cognitive impairment, poor environmental conditions, and traumatic experiences.

This leads us to commonly use the paradoxical intervention of *supporting the person's use of challenging behaviour when it is appropriate for their level of emotional development.*

In Jeremiah's case, it was noticeable that he did not receive any actual formal behavioural ('functional') assessment despite this being recommended by NICE. NICE (2015) states that there should be an individual, written behaviour support plan which includes 'strategies' that are 'proactive' and 'reactive'. This should be 'data driven', based on 'objective' action counts, and reviewed frequently, initially every fortnight. The assumption is that by increasing the 'skills' of family members, carers or professional care teams, they will not reinforce the challenging behaviour and instead only reinforce non-challenging behaviours. The guidance does not stipulate anything about the consistent availability of the carers, the need for their number to be small, nor anything about the quality of the relationship with the carer – certainly, nothing about their own attachment experiences or their caregiving behaviour from an attachment perspective.

Our experience continually challenges almost every one of these points. In fact, the 'data' often consists of incident reports that are poorly and inconsistently recalled; they tend to also be riddled with personal opinions and subjective comments. Reviews by behavioural practitioners and psychologists can approach or even exceed the two-week contact recommended by NICE, but attempts to impart behavioural skills are thwarted by staff turnover, rejection of the assessment by the carers, and the failure of this rather technical approach to resonate with the carers themselves, who view the person in terms of emotional transaction, not in terms of what they gain or avoid by way of their behaviour.

Recently, the only scientific trial meeting the 'gold standard' for research design failed to support NICE's position that simply training care staff on a behaviour support plan will significantly reduce or eliminate behaviours that other people find annoying or difficult (Hassiotis *et al*, 2018; Strydom *et al*, 2020). There is probably nothing technically wrong with the theory itself. PBS advocates such as David Allen and colleagues who actually provided the training in the trial have made a number of criticisms about the trials, such as them being based on a short-form of training involving three, two-day workshops, scepticism of some training recipients, poor 'homework' compliance, limited experience of some trainers, sporadic attendance by the care teams, and spontaneous recovery of some clients prior to entering the trials, and other practical issues (Allen *et al*, 2018). While they may have a point in saying that these problems with the delivery of the training may account for the lack of benefit to the people in the trial, these are all problems that clinicians face in their everyday practice when they try to deliver PBS, so there is no reason to assume that routine practice is any more effective than the trial suggests. Smaller studies which have supported PBS are less well-designed and prone to 'allegiance effects'[17]; it has to be noted that many of the authors who are

17 Results in the study are biased because the author wants their preferred approach to work. This can be unconscious and does not imply a lack of personal integrity, only a need for better-quality studies that can address bias.

trying to qualify or dismiss the findings of the Hassiotis trial will publish in journals that support the PBS philosophy (such as the *International Journal of Positive Behaviour Support*), and who are often personally invested in the success of behavioural approaches. It may be assumed that such advocates would be motivated to be very sceptical of evidence that challenges their favoured approach, given that the ineffectiveness of PBS is an existential threat to its widespread use as a clinical intervention.

Aside from the technical difficulties and – shall we say, generously – mixed evidence for viewing Jeremiah in terms of his behaviours that challenge, there is a more fundamental objection. Even if its evidence was overwhelming, we find that this approach rather misses the point. The symbolism of running away and the chaotic circumstances he found himself in were essentially rooted in his experience of early care and reflected how his family truly felt about him. This behavioural framework just seemed to reduce him to a collection of problems, a list of unwanted acts, even though it was presented with apparent compassion. Behavioural approaches never properly touch the emotional pain of other human beings, and never really address the processing of this pain; for Jeremiah, it was mainly trying to offer a way for other people to reduce any risk of physical harm, and to aim for his compliant quiescence. We would much rather have couched his case in terms of his emotional needs and experiences, whereby his actions can be seen as not particularly abnormal for someone in his situation. We found this to be much less 'othering' of Jeremiah – a behavioural model created a fundamental divide between everyone else on the one side, and him alone on the other – he had behaviours, whereas the rest of us have relationships[18].

Eventually, after about a year of meetings with little progress in the process of supporting Jeremiah with behavioural guidelines, the psychology team offered a different perspective following work in the organisation to prioritise trauma-informed care. It's important to state that, before the current trend across clinical practice for mental health to become more trauma-informed, it is unlikely that this approach would have been broached, given that it does not fit most of the narratives around people with intellectual disabilities who are described as 'challenging'.

18 I am grateful to Dr Beth Greenhill for this idea, which is paraphrased here.

Narrative 4: Jeremiah from a trauma-informed and attachment-based perspective (meeting 12 and beyond)

Readers might find it difficult to believe that, to start with, we could find no account of Jeremiah's early life experiences despite an extremely long clinical record. We therefore had to conduct an interview with his foster father, who had raised him since he was two years of age, in order to find out anything about his past. We kept in mind how he was currently seen as 'attention-deficient', 'intellectually disabled', 'depressed' and 'anxious', but we always assume that instead of being signs of a biological disorder, these are reasonable responses to the life a person experiences with the particular resources that they possess. We don't assume that problems with attachment are caused by poor parenting, though maltreatment is both more common in people with learning disabilities and also most commonly perpetrated by the family, at least when the person is a child. A relatively recent study that attempted to summarise the evidence of violence against children with disabilities in the English and Chinese-speaking worlds estimated that the risk is more than double, despite the growth in awareness of their particular vulnerability (Fang *et al*, 2022).

Looking at Jeremiah's case, he had experienced regular emotional and physical abuse from both his peers and his parents from a very young age. His father had been ill for many years with serious kidney disease, and his mother had periods of serious distress and even hospital treatment following several bereavements in her own family of origin before Jeremiah's fourth birthday. Due to their health issues, his parents could not earn enough money to look after all of their seven children, and they had trouble accessing benefits while being unwell due to changes in circumstances that kept altering their eligibility. Several of Jeremiah's siblings had been in prison due to antisocial and criminal acts. The senior school regarded Jeremiah as 'disruptive' and having variable motivation to learn, but they failed to consider what might be going on at home. They did regard him as 'anxious', but did not link this explicitly to times when he was being expected to be picked up from school by an uncle whose attendance at the school gates was patchy, often leading Jeremiah to be stranded at school until his father was called to pick him up when all the other children had left. Family members would argue with each other about who was responsible for Jeremiah, overtly trying to palm him off on each other. The message this conveyed was that he was not wanted.

The obvious link between multiple adversities and his underlying emotional state was never really considered as mediated by his unsatisfactory, intermittent and often hostile care from his family. One way of conceptualising this is by considering what happens in an anxious attachment relationship with a carer, as in the diagram below. The diagram suggests how a person would adjust or regulate their proximity to their nominated carer according to their anxiety, and the availability or otherwise of secure emotional care-giving,

Figure 13.1: Inhibition in learning and experiencing due to anxious attachment

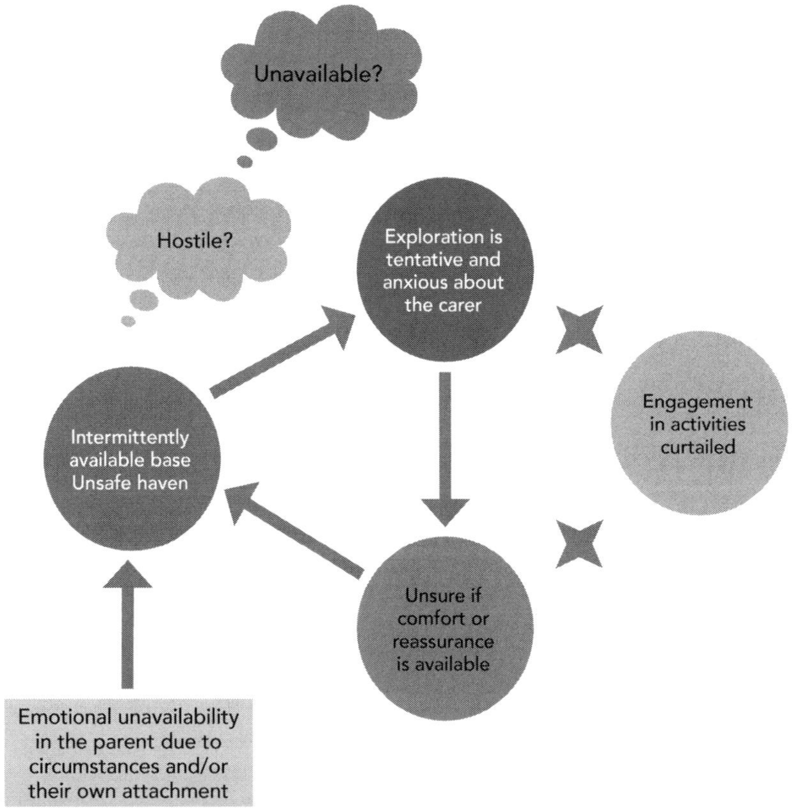

Since it was very difficult for professionals to name this poor parenting, no one wanted to do it before we became involved. This means that a trauma-informed formulation (a technical understanding) of the case had not been attempted. While the family's misfortunes were not their fault, they still had some responsibility and accountability for his presentation, and on the part of the professionals, there was a static, repetitive, almost compulsive tendency to just keep doing assessments and having meetings which created an illusion of activity in the absence of any real progress with him.

We generally dislike talk of 'leadership' in clinical teams, used as it is to promote people taking the role of directing *others* to provide effective interventions. In Jeremiah's case, there were no fewer than 18 people invited to his MDT meetings, of whom we estimated three to have any actual direct, personal contact. We consider this culture of having many leaders taking a consultative or supervisory role to be an organisational defence against face-to-face time with people in emotional pain. Jeremiah needed to be understood as needing consistent support in the form of a secure (unconditional and emotionally positive) approach to helping him explore the world, so that he would not be so worried all the time that he kept panicking about whether people actually cared or were just gearing up to reject or rebuff him. Running into shops and calling the emergency services indicated that his life was indeed characterised by emergency; at any time, he could be abandoned (emotionally or physically) or attacked by those who should have been kind and patient.

Professional meetings played into this process by promising some kind of help, but only resulted in professionals knowing him for a short time before passing on the case or simply avoiding him, possibly in the hope that someone else would confront the family about their shortcomings. Professionals do not like complaints, so they do not like to criticise each other in terms of their practice. Furthermore, campaigns are held within healthcare organisations that insist on the use of relentlessly positive language as ethical practice by their staff and which prioritises the need to value the opinions of carers over the need to take any kind of critical stance on their role in the person's life. It is therefore easy to go for the 'diagnose mental disorder and medicate' approach, as this takes responsibility away from the carers and prevents defensive complaints in response to criticism.

Sometimes this results in partial awareness of the organisational defences. Professionals can sometimes report conflicting reports in meetings within the same working week, one where there is a positive update, and one where there is a very negative one. One meeting reports that someone is moving house or care provider; another meeting is clear that this is not happening. Sometimes instances of professional input are reported as successful in one meeting, only for the team to hear that the placement is ending the very next day due to a crisis that was not reported in the previous meeting even though it had already occurred. This has been experienced as very confusing and frustrating by individual professionals, who talk about being perplexed or feeling like they are 'going mad' due to conflicting information.

The task was to stabilise his safety (by establishing a secure base) but this could not be acknowledged because of fear of retribution from his angry family. For the parents, *if only* a special boarding school, a special hospital, or a local authority home would meet Jeremiah's needs, then they could let him go without feeling guilty. For most of the professionals, if only he would respond to the medication, or the staff would follow the guidelines, or he would learn to regulate his emotions. For the advocate and the social worker, if only the professionals would get on with it (without knowing what 'it' was), then all would be well and his needs would be met, in some ideal way that had never occurred in his life as far as we could tell.

The truth is that no one wanted Jeremiah, in the way that people are joyously attracted to little children, or that one wants their romantic partner. No one lit up when they saw him. The family were all too preoccupied with their own needs and everyone was competing for very limited resources, emotional or otherwise. His preoccupation – which could be characterised as 'preoccupied attachment' or sometimes 'anxious attachment' – is an understandable response and, indeed, the sensible response, to being treated with scarce and intermittent affection. He seemed to feel a sort of starvation, which was reflected in his eating habits, where he craved enough to eat but rarely had it, resulting in looking very thin and drawn, so that there were several referrals to dietetics which did not result in any substantial intervention.

In psychoanalytic theory, it is sometimes said that clients who do not feel loved will struggle to eat enough because they must signal that they are unloved by showing people rather than using words. To speak of being unloved is unbearably painful, so concern is caused in others so that they will want to help and address the hunger. However, the person feels that, if they eat satisfactorily, they will be emotionally neglected again, so some people must keep restricting what they eat. This is often, if not always, accompanied by harsh criticism from self and others that their weight, body shape, fitness and appearance, which makes the person feel crushed and worthless. None of this need be conscious; indeed, it sometimes seems that it *must not* become conscious, as the explicit awareness that something crucial has not been provided would be emotionally overwhelming for both parent and child.

In partial support of this view, Adverse Childhood Experiences (ACEs) are indeed more commonly experienced by people who receive diagnoses of eating disorders (Rienecke *et al*, 2022).

We suggest that our team was prone to re-enacting Jeremiah's treatment by his family. Because no one addressed the interpersonal pattern, it simply happened again with the 'family' of professionals. Of course, proving scientifically that community services can act out the earlier relationships of people who are difficult to help with simple interventions is no easy task. Critics of psychoanalytic theory may even say it does not happen in this way, and that the mirroring of family dynamics with professional-client dynamics is coincidental or invented in the narrative created by people like us. We simply offer the idea in the hope that it might explain and extricate hard-to-support cases like Jeremiah's.

What interventions came out of using a trauma and attachment-focused approach?

We have engaged in several interventions with the organisation, the family and with Jeremiah himself. While we have attended the MDTs for him, and report our actions in this context, we consider that the meetings serve the psychological needs of professionals and the organisation, and in some ways, the family. They provide a way for professionals to discharge their responsibility to do something, for some form of process which they can appear to have worked within. However, we consider that the 'work' that is required is to develop an awareness that Jeremiah is treated in hostile and indifferent ways, and for him to be more adequately cared for in emotional terms. It is not simply a matter of confronting a family which is dealing with many stresses and strains, internal and external. This would only create a 'persecutor' role for us, in which we seem to be attacking others for not being good enough at being carers or professionals. The interventions we have carried out can be summarised as follows:

1. **Giving the context of emotional development.** We have assessed Jeremiah's emotional development and estimated that he has the emotional needs that are normally observed before attendance at primary school (18 months to three years, or 'first individuation'). We then provided an education session in combination with an accurate communication assessment from speech and language therapy to back up the findings of our assessment. This allows family and

carers to lower expectations of Jeremiah's ability to explore, engage in community activities and cope by himself, with more emphasis on being available to help him and accept that he cannot go out alone without becoming very anxious.

2. **Reducing the high number of carers and changeable care arrangements.** We have tried to influence the local authority to provide 'family-style' care in the form of a small care team, a home which he does not have to share with several other residents. We offered ongoing support to embed his assessment of emotional development into the expectations of new carers.
3. **An empathic narrative that is developmentally informed.** Via regular support sessions for front-line carers and his family, we introduced a narrative that asks others to respect his history. We reiterate that his 'challenging behaviours' are in fact *sensible responses to perceived threats* when he feels that he is being ignored, abandoned or overruled. They are developmentally normal, though appear abnormal to adults who do not know him, because of his physical size. When discussing or reporting on an 'incident', we ask that professionals reflect on how much demands for his compliance are a function of the inconvenience and embarrassment that others feel when he acts in ways that are not ideal for them. Does the matter feel urgent because someone is at actual risk of harm, which is unlikely? Does it just raise practical issues (how to find him, get him home)? We ask that he is not 'talked to' as though he can reflect calmly and rationally about 'managing' his own behaviour or 'self-regulating' his emotions. We also ask that any comments to him about an 'incident' are not punitive or disapproving and are instead aimed at understanding what he was feeling at the time.
4. **Challenging the use of powerful drugs that are very difficult to withdraw.** We raised the appropriateness of prescribing powerful mind-altering drugs, namely a drug developed ostensibly to treat depression, fluoxetine. The dose had been creeping up for several years, but this seemed only to sedate him when the dose was raised, and so it was dropped again. We felt that he should not be prescribed this medication because of the lack of benefit. This caused a serious disagreement with our medical colleagues, who felt strongly that it should not be reduced. We have been helped by our organisation's adoption of the STOMP programme (Stop The Over-Medication of People with intellectual disabilities). However, at the time of writing, a small reduction had

been reinstated due to withdrawal effects (as opposed to the 'return' of 'depression'), and worryingly, he has since been prescribed another powerful drug, Risperidone, which was developed to treat people experiencing serious disturbances in thinking such as hallucinations or serious delusions (although there is debate about whether such drugs are merely sedative rather than 'treating' the mental 'disorder'). This lack of progress, despite a clear steer towards a national programme of medication reduction/elimination, is very common in clinical services and continues to be an ongoing contention with different if not incompatible views being held even within the same community teams.

5. **Supporting direct interventions to help him express himself.** Instead of individual therapy, we collaborated with speech and language therapy colleagues to offer pointers on providing a safe base from which he could explore his world safely, engage with activities and seek support. We connected with two of his paid care team and advised on how to both prevent feelings of panic in public places and how to be reassuring, following the guidance that we developed in our emotional development training. While there were some printed materials and 'scripts' (a lot like the commonly used 'social stories'), this work was mainly about providing a feeling of empathy and understanding to Jeremiah's carers, so that their difficulties could be acknowledged. There were still times when no one knew what to do, but these were fewer and further between, and because we had undermined the 'social expectations' of 'good' behaviour, his carers were less stressed about these times. This created a benign circle.

Figure 13.2: Jeremiah's benign circle

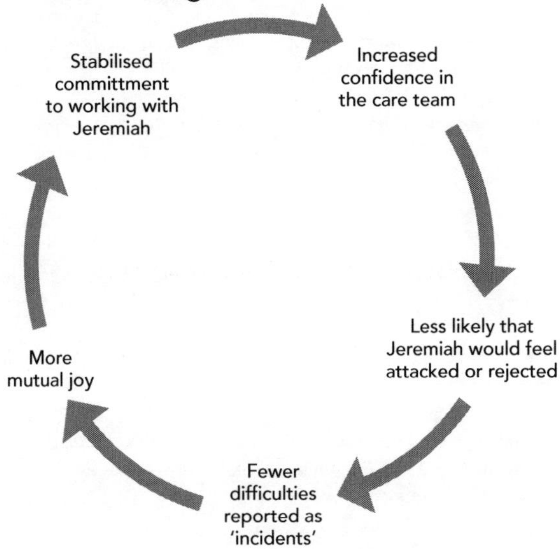

Looking back, that Jeremiah's improvement was due to our intervention is difficult to claim with scientific precision. The psychiatrist claimed that it was in fact the recent medication change that had caused the improvement. Without testing interventions in controlled conditions, it is not usually possible to work out what has helped, in clinical teams. This means that the *effectiveness* of our everyday work is not the same as claiming *efficacy* for a trauma and attachment-based approach. While we strongly suspect that it was taking a new approach that really helped Jeremiah, at the level of his own life experience, this is not the priority. What mattered is that he is more loved than ever – his life has times of safety, exploration, delight and comfort, and he can continue to experience ever-deepening bonds with his carers.

It is often surprising to the people we work with, professionals and carers, that we would see the development of love as both the job of the carer and the outcome we wish to see. It doesn't fit the professionalised language. But who is this language for? How does it help? Why is love rarely discussed when we are talking about caring for very vulnerable people? And why is it so rarely part of the equation when we know that insufficient love is at the root of a great deal of the suffering we see?

We deliberately leave these questions open for readers to consider.

References

Allen D, Jones E & Nethell G Clinical outcomes of staff training in positive behavioural support to reduce challenging behaviour in adults with intellectual disability: further thoughts on intervention, implementation and interpretation. *International Journal of Positive Behaviour Support*, **8** (1) 4-11.

Bion W (1961) *Experiences in Groups*. London: Tavistock.

Hassiotis A, Poppe M, Strydom A, Vickerstaff V et al (2018) Clinical outcomes of staff training in positive behavioural support to reduce challenging behaviour in adults with intellectual disability: Cluster randomised controlled trial. *British Journal of Psychiatry* **212** 161–168.

National Institute for health and Care Excellence (NICE) (2015) *Challenging behaviour and learning disabilities: prevention and interventions for people with learning disabilities whose behaviour challenges* [online]. Available at: www.nice.org.uk/guidance/ng11 (accessed September 2023)

Rienecke RD, Johnson C, Le Grange D, Manwaring J, Mehler PS, Duffy A, McClanahan S & Blalock DV (2022) Adverse childhood experiences among adults with eating disorders: comparison to a nationally representative sample and identification of trauma. *Journal of Eating Disorders* **10** (1) 72.

Skelly A, Shimmens V & Corner A (2022) Transforming nothing: the failure of the Transforming Care learning disability policy framed by the criticisms of Orwell's Politics and the English Language. *Clinical Psychology Forum* **350** 26-33.

Stokes J (1994) Problems in multidisciplinary teams: the unconscious at work. *Journal of Social Work Practice* **8** (2) 161-167.

Strydom A, Bosco A, Vickerstaff V et al (2020) Clinical and cost effectiveness of staff training in the delivery of Positive Behaviour Support (PBS) for adults with intellectual disabilities, autism spectrum disorder and challenging behaviour – randomised trial. *BioMedCentral BMC Psychiatry* **20** 161.

For more information on STOMP-LD, please see: https://www.england.nhs.uk/learning-disabilities/improving-health/stomp/

Chapter 14: Jonny

Criminal neglect

"The true character of a society is reflected in how it treats its children".

Nelson Mandela

This chapter describes a psychological therapy session with Allan Skelly provided to Jonny, a 30-year-old man who was referred almost incidentally for 'anxiety and depression' but was better known for his interactions with the police, courts and prison service. The recent death of his father, with whom he had become inseparable when not in prison, had not featured in his referral, which had asked for the psychology team to "educate Jonny that if he keeps offending, there will be bad consequences for him". He was the subject of a lot of professional frustration, was seen to be racist, paranoid about paedophilia, and was portrayed as 'a schizoid personality' (cutting himself off from others). He was also considered dangerous, due to a ten-year-old incident when he was arrested for assaulting a colleague at work, which had become central to his reputation.

Jonny arrived at the clinic for his fifth session. He was sitting with his hood up, avoiding eye contact. The administrators, behind safety glass, watched him carefully. His leg was shaking and he played with a lighter in his hands, turning it over and over. He looked up as I approached, saying, "It's me now, is it?" I noticed that this seemed very hostile in tone to those looking on[19]. As he got up to follow me, he appeared to kick the chair he was sitting on, and one of the administrators visibly flinched. Jonny smiled and said, "Oops".

We went into the therapy room. Jonny sat down and said, "Well, the doctor says I've got to stop eating chips because I am going to die, but I don't care, I've always had chips and I always have chips". I asked if he

19 The administrators had asked that Jonny not be seen by the team at the base, because they felt unsafe when he walked past them towards the therapy rooms. A risk assessment had determined that Jonny was at low risk of harming professionals, but I did empathise with their feeling, because an atmosphere of threat was present, at least initially. As to why he felt it necessary to create such a feeling in others, this will be explored.

was worried about his recent trip to see his family physician. He said, “Well, my dad’s dead, so what, eh?”

So, we were straight into the central issue of grief in the first moments of the session, but Jonny moved fast and before I could think of a response that might be of help to him, he asked, “So, why do you want to see me, what are you doing this for? I’ll tell you, it’s because you’re paid by Boris Johnson. I tell you what I want, I want someone to talk to me just because they want to.” I could not deny that I was paid to provide a therapeutic space. I said, “Well, it’s true I am paid to do this work, but you do deserve it; actually, you are entitled to it.” Jonny said, “Well, where in the f**k were you before I got in trouble?” He was starting to shout, and I imagined the admin staff calling the police and fantasised about the speech I would give them afterwards, about bark versus bite. Or, as Brett Khar (2021) has named, he uses insults (words) rather than spears (his fists), and so must have done some amount of self-healing. Somehow, Jonny had managed to rein in his anger and had been looking for someone to talk to for years.

This had not been offered. Identified as having a learning disability as a toddler, he had attended a special school, which was later found to have sexually, physically and emotionally abused the children systematically over several years. Jonny had never disclosed his own systematic sexual abuse until I had seen him. He had never told his parents what the teacher did to him. Furious that the perpetrator had only been sacked, not prosecuted, but unwilling to tell anyone about it, he had been seething with rage and the desire for vengeance for years. As often happens, he had been blamed and punished for the challenging behaviours that emerged from this abuse; fighting, bulling other children, refusing to work, absconding from school.

By this time in the therapy, Jonny had been able to verbalise his anger at authority figures for failing to protect him but was yet to see that we were re-experiencing this dynamic in our sessions. “What do you want, eh? Why do you want to see me? I just want to lock myself away from people. People are sh*t.” I asked if everyone was sh*t? He said, “Well no, my dad was alright. Not sure about you yet.” I said that it made sense to me. Why would he trust a world full of people who either violated him or didn’t help to stop it? He looked at me with a sudden quietness in his voice. “That’s right. Why bother? Why bother when all you get is accused? Accused of this, accused of that, accused of all sorts.”

It is difficult to describe in writing the change that occurred there. The attempt to understand rather than discourage, advise or rescue, altered the atmosphere from anger and danger to a deep and profound sadness. I could feel tears welling. It was as though I could see him as a child, vulnerable, doomed to horrible inescapable abuse for years and unable to find justice. I felt a pain in my chest and in my heart.

There had been one light in the darkness: his care for another little boy, who had childhood cancer, and whom he would accompany to school. He mentioned with uncharacteristic tenderness how his friend would wait with him at the bus stop, and he would wait at the window to see him coming up the road. At school, Jonny would push his friend's wheelchair and keep watch when the teachers were not present, and even at times when they were present.

Jonny said, "There's something more to tell you. You won't believe me, and you'll cover it up." Not knowing how to, or being unwilling to, negate my untrustworthiness, I simply waited for him to speak again. He continued, "I was raped at school. He used to come to the classroom and say, it's time for your physio. I would go because I thought I had to. He'd make me shower afterwards before bringing me back. Sometimes I was bleeding and I'd get in trouble later. I didn't even know it was wrong to start with." When Jonny finally complained about it, the member of staff simply disappeared overnight. There was no investigation, no police action, no interview. The abuse simply stopped.

Instead of relief, Jonny became convinced that he had done something else wrong. He didn't seem to have any moral reference point which could give him clarity about who was the perpetrator, who was the victim, and who was responsible. It was as though this was his lot in life, to be constantly the victim who was somehow to blame.

With bitter irony, Jonny had been prosecuted in his late teens, unsuccessfully, for sexual offences. Initially, this was mistaken identity in a case of exposure to members of the public, and the true perpetrator was later convicted. Jonny got a "half-assed, sh*t apology" from the police and prosecution service. He had then become known locally as a 'nonce' and an ex-partner accused him of multiple rapes. On all counts, he was acquitted, but obviously, this was an intensely traumatising and re-traumatising experience – to be accused of the very thing he had been repeatedly exposed to and had no justice for. He said, "You know when I think of it, I almost just walked out of that courtroom and killed someone. A member of the public. Just anyone, random like. I would have. I don't know why I didn't." I suggested that he had, through it all, never lost sight of right and wrong. I was still struggling with my own emotions. It was intensely difficult to bear what he was saying. I longed to talk about his difficulties in a recent review of benefits, or his diet; these were such soothing topics for us to discuss. I had done this in previous sessions, switching the topic, unconsciously wanting to deal with simple, practical matters; replace the chips with fried veg and the cola with caffeine-free, stop smoking, send his psychometric test results to the local council so that he could achieve a safe amount of financial benefit. Easy wins.

Prior supervision had caught my escapology. Jonny needed me to attend to the important things he was saying. I struggled, but eventually said, "You realise that everyone has been a child, and you really want to protect children". He became animated. "Where do all these f**kers come from? Why do they hurt kids? They should die. They should be tortured and put to death." Such thoughts tended to shade into his views on asylum seekers. "Like all those rapists in the channel. They are coming over here, they will get our women and children, given houses and all sorts." It was an invitation to argue. "You think I'm a racist, don't you? A scumbag." I said that I thought of him as someone who has had a life that taught him to look for threats, unfairness, things being taken away when they should not be... He interrupted; "My Dad said that! He said, you'll get no help, son. You're not one of them [immigrants/asylum seekers]. Don't ask for it."

Jonny felt safe with his dad, because his dad knew what to do or say when things were uncertain. He hadn't told Jonny about his cancer, and when he became very ill, still said he would get better soon. When he was released from juvenile custody at 18, Jonny and his dad had moved to the local area to get away from abusive associates, but in the process lost any network of friends that they had. Their life became very insular; visits to the shops or to their professionals or sitting at home. For Jonny, his life mostly revolved around gaming on his console, coffee and toast, with a simple meal in the evening. This was at least safe. The death of his father meant that he suddenly had to deal with being alone, as well as the funeral, paperwork, and the fundamental loss of his home as a safe place. This was not because his father was particularly loving; Jonny had basically been his father's carer in the last years of his life on a 24-hour basis, and would call out for him to change him, cook for him, and do all domestic tasks, at the expense of any kind of social life, romance or friendships.

It was no surprise that Jonny was cynical about my commitment to sufficient sessions. Since leaving custody just after his 19th birthday, he had been referred for help with his emotions on no less than 26 occasions, and each time he had attended, retelling versions of his story. This had resulted in some 14 detailed assessment documents but no intervention. Moreover, the assessments focused on his apparent risks to others, brief recommendations or signposting to voluntary services or online resources, and nothing focused on his abuse experiences, which were either ignored or quickly glossed over.

I said to Jonny that I was hoping to offer weekly sessions for as long as he needed. I hoped that this would be reassuring. He said "Why? What will you do? You think I am not worth anything. You think I am a racist." I said that it might seem strange, but I was more interested in why he had these thoughts and feelings. We'd focus on that, not on arguing or agreeing with him. He then said, "It's funny. I get something out of these meetings. I don't know what. I am a bit thick." The threat was gone. He seemed comfortable, and told me about his sisters, how they had gone to live in Mauritius and didn't bother with him. "I think one of them believes the girl who accused me – that I got off out of luck." This was despite the accuser being prosecuted for falsifying the allegations and other offences. "Why is it that when you are disabled and you want a girlfriend, you are a rapist or someone who gets raped?" He felt this dilemma to be real – all of his sexual experiences had been exploitative and cruel, and he was accused of being the perpetrator when, by any reasonable standard, he had been the victim.

I asked, "Has anyone ever treated you kindly, Jonny?" He couldn't think of anyone, then said, "There was none of this" and made a gesture as if taking a child in his arms, saying "There, there, honey. I didn't get any of that. I just got hidings if I did wrong. That's what I do. I lose my temper if someone walks into me looking at their phone. Or, if they get fed up with me in a shop if I don't understand. I get fed up and I shout. I knocked a guy at work out once because he kept saying that I was doing it wrong and losing the rag with me. Just slapped him and he fell over and I went home." This had become the defining act in Jonny's life. He became known in his records as someone who could suddenly, without warning or provocation, become violent. However, we were on the cusp of changing this.

"Would you treat a child in the way you were treated, Jonny?" I asked. "Never. I'd protect them and help them with their school and give them love and hugs. Every day." We had spoken about the idea of the inner child in previous sessions. "So, if you think of your inner child, they need someone to keep them safe, help them learn, and be kind when they are hurting. Could we do that here, in a way?" He looked at me, pensively. "Might do. Don't know. You could be trying to get something on me." He wanted to know if I would write anything down and who would see it. He said, "You know, this place is a bit like the youth centre where I was locked up while they called the police". I realised that the idea of a safe, contained time and place within a public service building, could be quite scary for him. It seemed to evoke feelings of somehow being in the wrong for simply feeling angry or vengeful. "But I would like to keep coming," he added quickly.

At the end of the session, Jonny suddenly looked at his watch, said, "Ah!", got up and walked out without saying goodbye. I was left feeling suddenly bereft and confused, which took a while to lift. It seemed that he was getting something from the sessions, but this was difficult to define in words. As I reflected on the session, I had an overwhelming feeling of loneliness, a feeling of being cut off from other people, as though his trauma was mine in some temporary way (transference). I felt the pull to care for his inner child within the 'therapy analogy', but also that he would find it difficult to accept, being as it was a challenge to his beloved father whose love was, at best, conditional.

An update on Jonny

Jonny has returned to sessions and made a solid commitment. He has made further disclosures of maltreatment as a child. We feel that he needs several years of psychotherapy in order to develop any trust in the outside world. Movingly – but unrealistically – he has said that the clinic is "the only safe place in the world" and has started to make tentative moves towards friendships that he finds mutually rewarding, safe and enjoyable.

Chapter 15: Constance

No one to let go of

"We are only as needy,
As our unmet needs."

John Bowlby, *Attachment and Loss*, 1969

This chapter is about Constance, a woman in her early 80s with only very limited language, mostly repetitive phrases. We were asked to 'analyse her behaviour' because she would struggle to share staff attention with the four other residents of her shared home, and staff were unable to complete their paperwork in the office. We do not describe the intensive behavioural interventions tried before we became involved, as they had not worked, but also we felt that the focus on her 'challenging behaviour' was functioning to hide deep feelings of dislike, even outright hatred of her. We describe our vain search for anyone with a kind word to say about her, and just how far a 'care team' can stray from empathy.

Constance was initially referred to us by her general practitioner following a request from her care team to 'give her something to knock her out a bit'. As often happens (and as seen elsewhere in this book), the medical model of disturbance or challenging behaviours is so strong in intellectual disability services that medications with little or no evidence are used widely, and it can be a shock for the care team when they are asked to modify their own behaviours and practices. This may even be considered critical of them, or offensive, and so alternative models have to be introduced with considerable training and support.

Constance's team had received many hours of behaviour specialist, physiotherapist, occupational therapist, speech and language therapist, and psychiatrist time prior to our involvement. Staff complained that she followed them around, repetitively demanded to go out to buy shoes, screamed when this was not possible or was seen as excessive, and asked repeatedly to be 'bandaged' on her left arm. She would throw paperwork in the air to prevent staff from sitting down to complete it and say, "Don't tell!"

We went to meet Constance and her care team, but on the day we attended she was asleep in her room. The door was open and she was being watched intermittently by staff who passed by. There were six staff on duty; two were doing laundry while talking about their family; three were sat in the lounge with Jerry, a man who was wheelchair-bound. Again, they were talking to each other and not talking to Jerry, although one person was feeding him a yoghurt, while turned around to talk to her colleagues. The final member of staff was Adam, who was the home manager. Adam asked us to sit in the office at the end of the bungalow – it was more of an industrial 'unit' than an actual house – and closed the door so that we could no longer see Constance. Adam was very keen to talk to us but was less keen on us observing Constance directly. He said, "Well, you won't be able to ask her anything, she only has a few words, a few compulsive words". He said that these words were "go out, buy shoes" and "look after my cuts and burns".

On questioning, the first of these was related to Constance's preferred activity, shopping. The second referred to her wish to be comforted and looked after through medicalised care. She would insist that staff take her to the first aid station and bandage her arm. She would appear most happy when walking home with new shoes (which may not be worn again) or when having her bandage done. If her carers refused or were busy, she would wail and scream, which would disturb the entire household and even cause other residents to become aggressive towards her.

As with many people like Constance, there had been extensive and repeated use of antipsychotic medication for most of her childhood and all of her adulthood, to try to reduce her 'agitation', presumably on the hypothesis that her behaviours reflected some kind of chemical imbalance in her brain, conceptualised in the historical notes as "schizoaffective disorder". While not as striking an example of polypharmacy as Jennifer (Chapter 16), we struggled to see how this diagnosis and the medication prescribed can have helped her, and there was little to no evidence that the changes and reviews of medication that resulted from appointments with various physicians had any effect on her behaviour, though it did seem to both disturb her sleep and her appetite when there were increases.

She had also received several referrals for behavioural interventions, but these were made by her medical staff, not her care team, who seemed somewhat bewildered as to why she needed a psychological approach. Their view was that this lady had a mental disorder (officially sanctioned as 'schizoaffective disorder') and her behaviours were therefore a kind of mania, due to problems in brain functioning. They felt that she should live in a hospital, where 'ill' people could be treated by medicine. Indeed, they frequently requested Mental Health Act assessments in the expectation that Constance would be taken to hospital, whenever her repetitive requests for shoes extended into the night and were accompanied by loud wailing. The meetings in which these requests were refused were uncomfortable and conflictual, with the commissioners, social workers and health professionals refusing to have Constance assessed under the Mental Health Act, and the care team saying that she was too ill for them, and they were worn out by her and did not understand her. She was simply "too unwell for us to cope with her".

Comprehensive trainings using a PBS model with strident input from psychologists, nurses, occupational therapists and speech and language therapists, occurred three times from 2015 to 2021. On each occasion of these thorough and detailed training events, entirely different staff seemed to appear, with the only constant being the presence of Adam. Following the second of these, which was two years after the first training event, Adam told us that a member of staff had been suspended and then sacked for allegedly locking Constance in a car having completely "lost it" after she had been wailing for several hours. We felt that this was likely to be the main trigger of the second referral to our team, as her behaviour seemed linked to the need to connect to someone caring, who would do something caring. Her requests to go shopping went down, and her requests to be bandaged went up.

While the Positive Behaviour Support process did eventually convince Adam that any behaviours of concern might reflect and underlying need to be stimulated and reassured, it did not focus on the 'who' of her care team at all. It was entirely focused on staff behaviours, as though the people involved were interchangeable. By carefully monitoring their activity plans, it could be seen that Constance's care was shared by more than 20 people, with a wide variety of personal mannerisms, views and concerns. Adam had identified that some staff were not as likely to experience long episodes of wailing, but these staff were seen as "giving into her" – meeting her demands for being taken to the kitchen, then to the laundry room, then to the bedroom, and sat down – and therefore should not be encouraged.

An alternative model was offered, since the PBS approach was clearly only temporarily effective, if at all. The new intervention was based around the idea of emotional development (see Chapter 2). A relatively brief assessment determined that Constance was functioning, emotionally, at the level of Socialisation (normally seen at the 6-18 months level). Demonstrating this level of emotional development brought into sharp relief the expectations of Constance versus her real needs. She could not communicate her actual needs using language, having only a few phrases that were used out of context and without easily understood meaning. She could take her care team by the arm if she wanted something, and despite advice to respond to this, many of her care team found this irritating and told her to "stop that". A particular difficulty was that it was not easy to know if Constance was unwell, as this led to lots of asking staff for food, which she would then throw down.

The emotional needs of a person in the Socialisation Stage can be shown as a modified version of the Four Tasks of Secure Caregiving diagram (see Figure 15.1). The person's priority is safety, which means they need to be constantly supervised while awake, to prevent injury and distress.

In order to provide a secure base, it is necessary for Constance to feel that people are trying to interpret her signals, and this is difficult and imprecise, as with all people at that level of functioning. She needs more or less constant attention from the carer. To help her explore, her carers need to tolerate some frustrated lashing out, and interests that are too intense to be adaptive in themselves but have a sensory value (the shininess of shoes being her interest), but they are also empowered to limit such purchases, as the model clarifies fully that such 'choices' cannot be underpinned by mental capacity[20].

As such, her care team needed to become more directive and to provide her with structure. We therefore encouraged limited shopping trips but also introduced alternatives that would meet Constance' interest in shiny objects by providing sensory materials and these being rotated from a 'sensory library' so that the novelty could also be experienced. We also pointed out that staff could use light tones and high voices as they would

20 Indeed, previous attempts to enhance 'choice', based more on equality principles and her chronological age, can be seen as unwittingly oppressive, in that she simply refused many options because she did not understand what was being asked of her. It was a marked change in her life circumstances for outings and activities to be planned by her care team, and even though she would initially resist activities, her overall experience of them became much more positive, with knock-on benefits to her evenings, sleep patterns and appetite.

Figure 15.1 How to provide a secure base, exploration, engagement and comforting / reassurance at the 6-18 month level of emotional development (socialisation stage)

16-18 Months Emotional Development

This is when Attachment Patterns appear in children's development.

They have to **feel safe to explore.**

1. Create safety:

Being closely available to prevent accidents.

Meeting personal care needs from 'signals'.

Using constant warm tone.

Recognising and responding to emotions (but don't expect the person to name or comment on feelings).

2. Promote exploration:

Providing the structure and activity plans.

Providing different environments e.g soft play, swimming pool, but with the same adults where possible.

Encouraging exploration of the immediate environment with toys.

Remembering that choice is not a priority.

Expecting frustration and some 'defiance'.

No need to seek 'peer' settings yet.

Remain close to prevent accident (falls, burns, head bangs etc.).

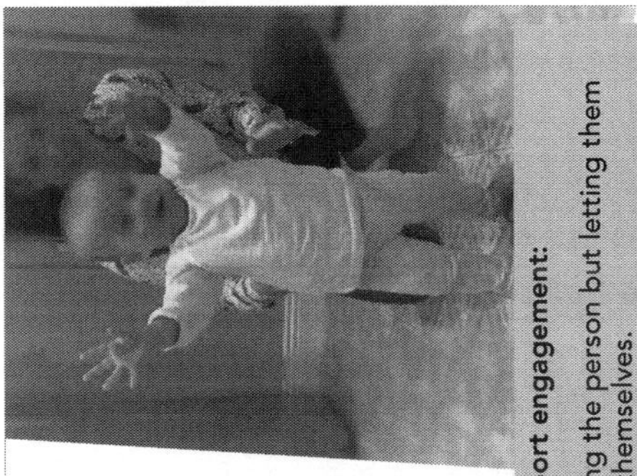

3. Support engagement:

Following the person but letting them act for themselves.

Activities remain props for relating, not skills learning.

Positive joint attention: i.e. make eye contact to the person, then to the object or activity, then positively vocalise, then return gaze to them.

Delighting in any 'discovery'/happiness or contentment.

Expecting only brief attention to an object before continuing exploration.

4. Provide comfort and reassurance:

Addressing physical discomfort immediately.

Keep eye contact while reassuring the person.

Talk in a reassuring tone without expecting formal understanding of what you say.

Considering what was distressing the person.

Doing the thinking for them as a 'unit'.

SOCIALISATION
SAFETY SEEKING

with young children. This was not 'patronising' (they feared being seen as talking down to Constance), and coincided with a marked improvement in their understand of her.

Unfortunately, the care team was affected greatly affected by the COVID outbreak, both in terms of limited access to the community and staff illness.

An Update on Constance

The issue became complicated because the team did not know how to explain the sudden absence of the person, Jackie, whom Constance had been very focused on. When we visited, dressed as we were in gloves, masks and aprons, we found to our disappointment that there was an entirely new team. Adam, following a bout of stress, had taken a new job and didn't work a notice period. The new manager, Ann, made it clear that this was just a change at the professional level and that if we just retrained them in behaviour management techniques, they were hopeful that Constance could be dealt with. In response, we summarised our involvement and tried to explain the ideas we had been developing with Constance's previous team.

We often find it demoralising to work with systems that can suddenly replace all of a person's social network, without seeming to perceive the emotional impact of this. Especially in the light of Constance's level of emotional development, the impact of these changes can only be seen as complex bereavement. Coupled with this, the introduction of ideas about very limited emotional development and the attachment needs that a person has in the light of this limited development, clashes with the service philosophy and workforce economics in the care sector.

In the end, just before her death in 2022, Constance had no deep, enduring bonds with anyone. She was remembered within our own team as a person whose funeral was not attended by anyone who knew her well. We wondered whether her care manager, professionals and new care team simply felt relief at her passing. It was extremely painful to meet her and feel how lonely she looked, even in a seemingly busy bungalow. Does anyone miss her, mark her memory, or feel any fondness in retrospect? And even if there was some affection somewhere, where is the memory of her as a child, a babe in arms, someone's gorgeous baby? This is perhaps the least-known but profound aspect of her life – that there was no one to let go of. In her life, 'care' only existed as a word on a page. There was no one who loved her, no one who looked into her eyes and said, "You are lovely", no delight, no fun, no laughs; just demands to be compliant and non-challenging, beyond her capability to comply.

Chapter 16: Jennifer

Labelled to death

"Labels are for filing. Labels are for clothing.
Labels are not for people".

Martina Navratilova

This chapter describes Allan Skelly'ss investigation into the lost life history of Jennifer, which he carried out in the last year of her life. She had developed a degenerative condition, irreversible Tardive Dyskinesia, following many years of 'treatment' with multiple drug regimes. Allan found the chaotic, random and often unresponsive nature of her medical care to be extremely disturbing. Not only did Allan consider that many of her 'symptoms' were known side effects of her medication, but also her traumatic history was completely avoided; there were many professionals in her life, but no one wanted to consider that her 'challenging behaviours' were responses to being drugged, ignored and periodically assaulted.

Jennifer was an elderly woman with an apparent severe disability, who had lived for 40 years in a long-stay hospital, whom we met at age 55, having finally been moved into a two-bedroom home when the institution closed.

We were asked to see Jennifer and her care team to address, of all things, attempts to steal telephones from members of the public during outings into the community. It was the first time we had come across the idea of kleptomania as a formal diagnosis. Jennifer would grab the phone, run away as fast as possible for a short distance, and then throw the phone down. Previous work had identified that she had this tendency and should have her access to the local shopping precinct limited, and eventually, community visits were stopped altogether. It was said that, "She might hit a child when she throws the phone". Strangely, her consultant psychiatrist had also asked the current staff team to consider allowing open access to their mobile phones in the home, to prevent challenging behaviour.

We were invited to a large multidisciplinary meeting held at her home, where we were made very welcome with tea and biscuits. On the way in, we asked to look in on Jennifer. She sat in a large armchair, and she looked up and said hello, then looked away, laughing softly. She seemed not to really be 'present'. It was as though meeting someone new meant very little to her.

As we were shown into the meeting, there were many jokes and discussions of people's various lives, holidays, social events, their journey to the home, and the poor phone reception (Jennifer lived in a very rural location, with very few local services). The community nurse, social worker, psychiatrist, neurologist, and even the family doctor were present. Tea, coffee and various biscuits and snacks were provided and consumed with good humour by the visiting professionals. We joined in and had a drink and a biscuit. It seemed quite the 'party', and the uniqueness of so many professionals attending for a person with a learning disability struck us strongly. This has never happened since and had not happened before. On reflection, I noticed that no one was talking about Jennifer, or how she was, perhaps because no one had the answer to the 'challenging behaviours'. Jennifer was described as 'aggressive', but on questioning, this involved occasional outbursts, mainly at night, which never became physical, and having crying episodes when being helped in the toilet. The original complaint, taking phones from other people in the community, had faded completely from view.

Eventually, some 20 minutes into the meeting, some discussion started to occur about Jennifer. Initially, this was very focused on her physical health, including seizures, the need for dental extractions, and her blood sugar. There was also a lengthy discussion about her refusal to have her blood taken, which was rather dangerous because she was receiving the powerful drug lithium, which can be very toxic.

While we had been told that it was 'essential' for a psychologist to attend the meeting, no one began a conversation about Jennifer's psychological needs. The main focus was on her going to hospital for investigations. While she definitely would be seen as 'lacking capacity to consent to medical intervention' and therefore could be – for want of a better word – *forced* to go, no one seemed willing to make the decision. It had to be a vote. We became voters in a decision taken on someone's behalf – usually called their 'best interests' – which is generally the only time someone can make a healthcare decision for another person unless there is a previous handing over in what is called an Enhanced Power of Attorney.

Somewhere in the collective mind of this group, there was anxiety; anxiety about getting it wrong. The current diagnosis was potential Alzheimer's disease, as she seemed to be losing skills she had shown previously (though these skills were never well specified). She was more distressed, and would often sit by herself, wailing. Occasionally, Jennifer would be heard to make disconcerting vocalisations in the night, such as "Doctor, doctor!", and "Get you!", "Police!", "It's illegal!" or "No, no!" These 'outbursts' were interpreted as signs of psychosis by several professionals, requiring 'medication review' by some professionals, and by others as seeking attention. No one seemed to consider that these might be memories of maltreatment and that attention to her might be appropriate.

Looking back on this meeting afterwards, I had experienced guilt that I could not speak up against all of the 'biologism'. It was too easy an explanation, but it also raised uncomfortable issues. No one was considering her life as a series of experiences, or even in any sense considering her history, even the history of medication use. Our assistant psychologist, Esme, later undertook to get all of Jennifer's files out of the archive to construct some kind of timeline, so that we could get a better sense of what had happened to her.

As an infant, Jennifer had struggled to feed, did not smile, and there were concerns expressed by health visitors and social workers about her being 'unresponsive'. Jennifer's parents described 'tantrums' and 'rage', not witnessed by professionals, and felt that they could not cope with her disability. After discussions between paediatricians and her parents, she was admitted to a special hospital for what was called Permanent Care at the age of five years. It was not long before she was diagnosed with 'hyperkinesis' (aged seven), mania (aged nine), schizophrenia (aged 11), schizoaffective disorder (aged 14), then bipolar disorder (aged 20), then later, Parkinsonism (aged 40 – but it was recorded that this was a primary diagnosis, rather than an obvious effect of long-term use of strong psychoactive drugs).

Each of these diagnoses was made with great confidence and was associated with a particular medication. As a young child, she was put on stimulants (methylphenidate – 'ritalin') for hyperkinesis (not being able to concentrate for long), which was adjusted regularly without much effect. For her 'mania' (being very active and crying – described as 'manipulative wailing' – to the nursing staff) she was given thioridazine[21] and carbamazepine at alarmingly high doses. Later, she was placed on olanzapine for the supposed 'schizophrenia', which was largely diagnosed because of her apparent dissociated memories, which, when stated to the nursing staff, was taken as evidence of 'voice hearing' hallucinations. However, there was never any convincing evidence of hallucinations, and even if there had been, olanzapine and similar 'antipsychotics' do not act against hallucinations directly, rather they lower anxiety for many people who are acutely and severely distressed – and then the symptoms gradually become less frightening. They are probably helpful for short-term use, but because of the common and serious side effects of withdrawal, many people end up on them long-term, or even for life[22].

Eventually, because Jennifer refused to comply with nursing staff and would frequently take extra drinks that were outside of 'hospital drinks time', she was considered to be 'hypomanic' and later to have 'bipolar disorder', causing her to be placed on lithium.

Olanzapine and carbamazepine continued to be administered despite their powerful effects on her condition. She became more passive, but still was prone to lashing out during her personal care, especially when washed in sensitive areas by staff who did not know her very well.

Looking at the clinical notes, Esme was surprised, and we were not a little alarmed, that the 'evidence' for the introduction of each medication was anecdotal opinion of a particular nurse or nursing assistant, in short 'clinics' and 'clinical discussions' with psychiatrists who visited the ward. Often the nursing staff barely knew Jennifer; the ward used a lot of agency or 'bank' staff rather than a small group of staff who would know her better. The psychiatrists, too, were often rotational trainees, schooled in the biological theory of mental illness. They would pick up the current working idea, e.g., that she was bipolar, without reviewing all of her history and questioning the diagnosis critically (this would not have

21 Thioridazine was globally withdrawn in 2005 when it was found that it could cause severe heart arrhythmia. Jennifer had been administered it for several years and was only (slowly) taken off it when the dangers became public. Prior to its withdrawal, the consultant psychiatrist had repeatedly rejected family requests for it to be reduced, saying this was too dangerous, again, using the "insulin for diabetes" metaphor.

22 See joannamoncrieff.com and the critical psychiatry network to find out about the disputed mechanisms of 'antipsychotics' and 'antidepressants'. The names themselves are actually developed from marketing practices with the support of psychiatrists who support biological explanations of psychosis; previously, antipsychotics were called "major tranquilisers", a term that more accurately describes their action.

been very wise when one wants a positive evaluation from the consultant psychiatrist). Changes would then be made as though they were the first time anyone had prescribed anything to her.

The final major change to medication came at the age of 52, when she was briefly given the drug Levodopa to address the apparent development of Parkinsonism. This was an even more contentious issue, as we were convinced that the Parkinsonian symptoms (freezing for periods of time, then having expansive 'choreiform' movements and being very active) were in fact signs of Tardive Dyskinesia, a permanent and debilitating syndrome that results from side effects of drugs like olanzapine. This medication was quickly stopped when Jennifer was reported to become 'very angry'. No one ever considered that she might be trying to express her frustration and that the Levodopa may have opened a window on her feelings, just as was depicted in the film *Awakenings*.

So, there we were, invited into the life of a person who, from early childhood, had been considered to have an elusive but pervasive disease of the brain. In her clinical records, she was never described in terms of the working relationship with her care team; it was as though she was not a person, she was a clinical phenomenon, an epileptic-attention-deficient-schizophrenic-parkinsonian entity with no personhood.

There was one professional who stood apart from the biological model and the pharmacological approach, without overtly challenging it. The speech and language therapist, Camilla, was very committed to *Intensive Interaction* as an approach to working with non-verbal people. Intensive Interaction involves many of the skills that loving parents will show their infants, by making eye contact, smiling, vocalising in a way that 'takes turns' with the child, and using the 'burst-pause' method of holding attention for a time. Recipients learn that those who care for them will 'be there', delight in their very existence, and thus develop feelings of agency and internal value. Camilla had even proved its effectiveness by showing in video analysis that Jennifer was much more responsive, lively and showing signs of pleasure (smiles and cooing) when she was doing an Intensive Interaction session, and showed fewer behaviours that others considered challenging.

By contrast, 'control' (comparison) observations showed that she would sit alone and self-stimulate by rubbing herself or masturbating. Her world was rather unpredictable; she could never tell when staff would approach to replace her continence pads or take her to the bathroom. She was often clearly thirsty, and her diet was poor. Her 'choices' to eat very unhealthy foods were, strangely, seen as informed, so Jennifer was obese. Her reticence, due to imbalance, to go out like she used to was seen as agoraphobia and part of her Parkinsonism. She was described as a "difficult client" because "it is hard to know how to please her".

However, we felt strongly that this was not a fair view of Jennifer's presentation. When we applied Došen's stage model of development by way of a *Scale of Emotional Development*, it was found that Jennifer had never really developed beyond the first stage of emotional development, *Adaptation*. Typical of the first year of life, in Adaptation, the person has no sense of any difference between the caregiver and themselves and cannot differentiate between strangers or familiar people in any clear way – they must get to know their parent or carer over time, through familiarity. It is extremely important that care is tailored towards an absence of pain, discomfort or cold. It is also important that the person is constantly attended to, which can be very tiring for the caregiver if they must balance this with their own self-care, work, etc. Communication is non-verbal, and behaviours that are distressing to observe, such as self-injury, should be seen as an appeal, the expression of a need that is not being met. Needs should be met without delay. The person cannot be 'spoiled' – this very idea should be jettisoned as it is unhelpful and unjust. While it might be difficult to know how to respond to every vocalisation, because the person has a very limited range of signals (often crying or 'wailing'), the caregivers should have a list of caregiving actions to try – typically the removal of discharged fluids, the provision of satisfying food, the adjustment of ambient temperature, and the provision of gentle, limited stimuli. The person may not respect the expected downtime, having no sense of night or day. Stereotyped movements – rocking, hand-flapping, or masturbation – are not merely self-stimulation, they are a coping mechanism for states of tension and indicate that the person is not adequately attended to. The person is very susceptible to the emotional 'atmosphere'. There is 'emotional contagion', i.e. distress in the carer is a normal response to the person's signals that they are uncomfortable and in need of help. It is important to acknowledge this as part of the caring work, and for carers not to be 'cut off' (with or without the justification of being 'professional').

By taking this framework to understand Jennifer, there is not (and never was) any need to add a mental disorder or other diagnosis to explain why she was considered a difficult person to care for as she grew up. To her very limited emotional development was added separation from her parents, institutionalisation, living in a large group ward (rather than a small family setting), and then suddenly having to move later in life because of policy changes (rather than because it was what she needed, personally). Within a model of emotional development, the appropriateness of her initial admission, the necessity of the various diagnoses she was given – and, by extension, the strong medications, and even the idea that her behaviour was 'challenging', all come into question. Her living situation, for most of her life, did not allow anyone to love her in the way that a parent loves a child in the first year of life, but that is what she needed.

The behavioural model, as applied by the behaviour specialist nurse involved in the case, provided indirect evidence of the above as well. In specifying, recording and counting incidents of vocalisations, self-injury in the form of slapping herself, and occasionally slapping or biting others, it was found that she would either want to avoid discomfort (e.g. when her pad was wet or soiled) or over-stimulation, (e.g. long days out), or gain the attention and interaction with staff. While a behavioural assessment tends to identify social interaction as a 'function' of challenging behaviour – and thus implies that it is an acceptable human need – it says little about the emotional bonds between the carer and the cared-for. The recommendations made – for example, that she should have Intensive Interaction at structured times of the day, access to a sensory box, music time, removal of triggering noises, etc. – were all 'depersonalised'. They can be delivered by anyone, be they someone who has known her for 20 years, or an agency nurse on their first day working with her.

We feel that it is incredibly naïve to create 'care' that is depersonalised in this way, without regard to the need for people with limited emotional development to have a small number of consistently available carers. While many practitioners promote 'consistency', they often mean consistency in following behaviour support plans, with each carer or support worker following the instructions of the plan. We know, however, from the idea of *object constancy* that prolonged separation and impermanence in caring relationships can be very damaging, if not traumatising.

Object constancy refers to an understanding that the relationships we rely on are stable, hopeful and intact, even though the other person frustrates us. In early childhood, this is based on the concept of object permanence (knowing that if our mother or father leaves the room, they still exist). While we lack object constancy, being left alone can cause feelings of terror, which is often argued to be rooted in a deep human fear of abandonment. Jennifer had not only been moved from the relative consistency of her family to institutional care but was then cared for without the special and devoted attention that each child deserves. It follows that she could be expected to become 'overactive' to gain the the scarce attention of the staff who had very limited time for each patient in the hospital. It cannot be assumed that even these brief moments of care were kindly or warmly provided; such hospitals could be chaotic and cruel, with low staff morale, poor leadership, and little scrutiny of what passed for 'care'. More desperate acts to obtain some kind of interaction or agency might, of course, be considered 'manic'. Using her single-word utterances, Jennifer resisted unspecified instances of theft and violations of her bodily space that were both sanctioned (such as medical examinations) and unsanctioned (such as alleged attacks and unwanted sexual advances). A lot of abuse of people with learning disabilities remains unknown (Sullivan & Knutson, 2000), and large institutions were notorious for this hidden, sorry phenomenon.

When Jennifer was in her 20s, she started to show apparent interest in nudity, but would also be angry while trying to touch and undress staff and other patients. This was described in her notes as "evidence of bipolar disorder in the form of disinhibited behaviour". No one seemed to consider why a young woman, often unsupervised and unable to relate any assaults upon her person, might suddenly show sexualised, angry behaviour. It is known that the start of inappropriate sexualised behaviour is a sign of sexual abuse in those showing such behaviours (Beail & Warden, 1995). Yet, with Jennifer, any behaviour change was seen as evidence of a mental illness.

Let's just pause here to consider what we have described. A child who could not behave as expected was placed, at an early age and even earlier stage of emotional development, into an impersonal institution that neglected her need for attention, interpreted her actions as signs of a mental illness requiring drug treatment, and probably failed to protect her from sexual and physical abuse. She was given strong psychoactive medications in order to address the perceived abnormality of her behaviour, in the absence of any consistency or rigour in the proposed mental illnesses that were cited as the reasons for drug use.

Without anyone she could consider a parental figure, Jennifer had to develop some way of meeting her need for human contact and stimulation. We considered that her attachment behaviour, if we can call it that, approximated this diagram:

Figure 16.1: The problem of conflating a person with psychiatric diagnoses

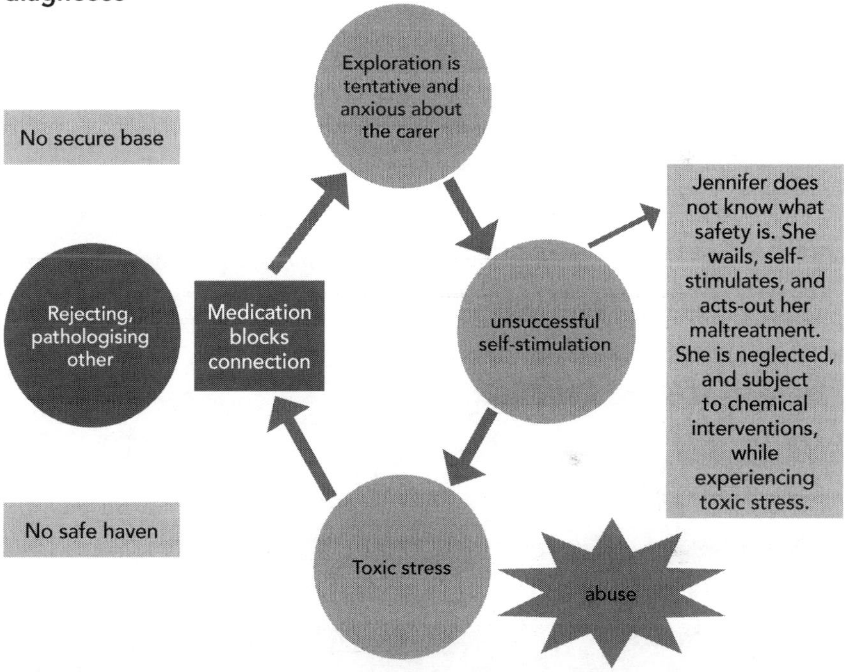

Jennifer had been on a wide range of drugs that alter brain chemistry. Many people think that these drugs are not like illegal drugs or alcohol; it is often assumed that they act like 'insulin for diabetes', and that this is why people have to take them for life. However, this idea has been debunked and is now not even claimed by psychiatrists, who still maintain that diagnoses such as schizophrenia are 'brain diseases', or the pharmaceutical industry, who will obviously have some investment in the idea that their products are necessary.

Once we are understood as a "person with schizophrenia" for example, this creates a reduced understanding of the person we are, as a person with a physical condition, with an implied neurological basis. It therefore follows that a chemical, or even surgical, intervention might somehow stop our brain from causing our distress to be so unbearable. The chemical interventions for schizophrenia were long held to correct a 'dopamine imbalance' (the dopamine hypothesis). While the theory has been debunked by careful research on post-mortem brains (Moncrieff, 2009), the drugs that are supposed to correct this imbalance are still regularly prescribed on the basis of their alleged benefits (which are themselves contested). This means that there is no clear mechanism of action for many of the current, licenced drug treatments.

"Antipsychotic medications have been used to modify ... behaviours in people with a learning disability, but there is little evidence to suggest that the benefits outweigh the risks."

Brylewski & Duggan, 2004

And what are these risks? Let us consider just one of the medications that Jennifer was made to take for more than 20 years, olanzapine.

According to the company producing it, olanzapine has no fewer than 18 side effects that commonly occur:

- akathisia (an inability to sit still)
- constipation
- headache
- dizziness
- light-headedness
- drowsiness
- tiredness
- restlessness
- weight gain (more likely in teenagers)
- increased appetite
- memory problems
- stomach pain or upset
- loss of bladder control
- back pain
- pain in arms or legs
- numbness or tingly feeling
- breast swelling or discharge (in women or men)
- dry mouth
- missed menstrual periods.

However, within the provided medication information, there can be found over 40 serious side effects, including:

- uncontrolled muscle movements in your face (chewing, lip-smacking, frowning, tongue movement, blinking or eye movement)
- trouble speaking or swallowing
- swelling in the hands or feet
- confusion
- "unusual thoughts or behaviour"
- hallucinations

- thoughts about hurting yourself
- sudden weakness or ill feeling
- fever
- chills
- sore throat
- swollen gums
- painful mouth sores
- pain when swallowing
- skin sores
- cold or flu symptoms
- cough
- feeling very thirsty or hot
- inability to urinate
- heavy sweating
- hot or dry skin
- upper stomach pain
- itching
- loss of appetite
- dark urine
- clay-coloured stools
- yellowing of the skin or eyes (jaundice)
- increased thirst
- increased urination
- hunger
- dry mouth
- fruity breath odour
- drowsiness
- blurred vision
- weight loss
- very stiff muscles
- high fever
- confusion
- fast or uneven heartbeats
- tremors
- light-headedness.

How could Jennifer have reported these effects, should they have occurred? It would take a great degree of observer interpretation in many instances, with the ongoing risk that the side effects could be interpreted as ‘challenging behaviours’. Remember, Jennifer was initially referred for grabbing phones from members of the public. Was this perhaps because of olanzapine-induced confusion, or even just to draw attention to her distress? In the side-effect list are the very symptoms it is intended to reduce – hallucinations and “unusual thoughts and behaviour”.

Living with even mild side effects can be horrible. For example, akathisia is an inability to remain physically still. People who feel it describe feeling tense and uncomfortable, and unable to sit still. They rock, shift feet and pace when standing, and struggle to remain seated. To feel like this because of a medication that is intended to calm a person and relieve distress seems almost perversely ineffective.

When Jennifer started to show signs of Parkinsonism, there was much debate among professionals as to whether it was drug-induced or not. As is expected, the consideration of whether this was the case was left to the medical personnel who continued to recommend the use of the medications. A consultant neurologist who had reviewed Jennifer had, several years before we were involved, deferred to her psychiatrist because of how many drugs Jennifer was administered. It was almost as though she had a second meal consisting of pills at breakfast and dinner. At the time the Parkinsonism was diagnosed, and it was stated that this was nothing to do with her drug regime, she was on pregabalin (to reduce 'anxiety'), fluoxetine (to address 'depression'), olanzapine (to address 'aggression'), lithium (to address 'mood swings'), and over-the-counter painkillers for when it looked like she was in pain. She also had to have drugs that prevented her psychoactive drugs from upsetting her stomach. We could never quite shake the feeling that the drugs were a substitute for acknowledging that she was emotionally neglected, lonely and desperately in need of comfort. Administering them made the nurses feel better.

What would our understanding of Jennifer be?

Alternative models do exist and may be more aware of trauma, institutionalisation, and in particular, emotional neglect. For example, the *Power Threat Meaning Framework* from the British Psychological Society (Johnstone & Boyle, 2018) is a way of understanding psychological distress from a perspective that emphasises that most of what upsets us is due to what has happened to us (rather than what is 'wrong' with us). Our own formulation (a tentative summary explanation of why Jennifer presented as needing help) would have been something like this:

In the late 1960s, a child experienced a physical event which affected her brain as an infant or small child; the main candidate was an infection when she was 18 months old. This had cognitive effects that the family struggled to adjust to. Her parents were distressed by how she seemed to be developing, not walking at the expected times, and they did not know how to help, so they sought the advice of medical professionals. On meeting the family, a paediatrician recommended that Jennifer be placed in the Permanent Care of the Local Special Hospital for the Mentally Handicapped[23]. They were unsure but agreed to sign the papers.

Jennifer did not settle well into the hospital. She found it frightening and missed her family. She lived in a large dormitory which was understaffed and had little to do during the day except to go for a walk in the large grounds or take part in domestic tasks, which did not interest her. Drinks were delivered communally on a large tray and meals served in a large dining room in a way that one sees in some schools. Aggression between patients was commonplace and usually unreported. Some other patients were extremely aggressive and disturbed, frightening Jennifer further. As her body developed, she became a target for sexual assault.

This institution did not encourage strong bonds with the staff, and often used punitive methods to control behaviour throughout the 1970s and into the 1980s. Jennifer was subject to a programme of reward through token economy for using quiet vocalisations, but if she was considered to 'wail' for more than 30 seconds she was subject to 'time out' (secluded until she stopped). This was based on a psychologist's assessment that she was seeking attention by wailing. In straight contradiction of what attachment theory suggests about this kind of 'appeal', Jennifer was instead subject to a cruel and perverse conditioning to need less and less interaction with other people. When she did show her need for interaction, her medication and her current diagnosis would be reviewed, often leading to additional medications.

No one ever considered whether her need to seek out others to meet her need for basic care was appropriate for her stage of emotional development, nor did they consider if some of the stranger actions, like stealing drinks, were side effects of her being subject to strong psychoactive substances over long periods of time. She was left somewhere between an Avoidant attachment pattern, where she did not approach the staff for fear of hostility, rejection or coldness, and Disorganisation of attachment, where such figures are actually feared.

Was Jennifer 'labelled to death'?

Meeting Jennifer was a sad experience. She was obviously wary of us, as she was of all professionals. Only Camilla had any real rapport with her,

23 This was prior to the *Better Services for the Mentally Handicapped* White Paper of 1972, which started the long and arduous process of de-institutionalisation.

but it is a sign of how resilient our underlying tendency to seek connection can be that Camilla was able to achieve this in what was previously a wasteland of utter loneliness.

Her care team in her last home, after de-institutionalisation, observed Camilla at work and formed a kind of 'distant fondness' for this 'mysterious' lady who avoided them, but occasionally shouted abuse at them or cried softly in her bed or on her sofa. As the neurological effects of Parkinsonism took hold, she started to spend long periods frozen to the spot, seemingly unable to move, tears rolling down her cheeks. We visited, but apart from a few golden moments with Camilla, there was little to feel positive about. It made us determined to tell her story, so that in some small way, it could prevent what happened to her from happening to others.

Jennifer finally passed away about two years after she was diagnosed with Parkinson's. Her family did not want any professionals to attend the funeral, so we had a small get-together as a team to toast her over coffee and cupcakes. Camilla told everyone about her work, which was clearly the highlight of the team's work with Jennifer.

Of course, in our role as psychology professionals, we could never prove that her medications directly shortened her life, but equally, we noted that she developed Parkinsonian symptoms after many years of exposure to strong drugs associated with this syndrome, without (in our view) clear evidence of 'psychosis'. Jennifer had relayed and acted out what appeared to be memories of being inappropriately touched while an in-patient, and these memories seemed to play out like a film script in a way which people who have post-traumatic symptoms would clearly recognise. People with intellectual disabilities are consistently over-medicated, often with powerful drugs intended for the acute treatment of people who develop serious delusional beliefs that could cause them to harm themselves or others, or severe and distressing hallucinations. It was never established that Jennifer had any coherent syndrome involving these symptoms. The medical staff in the institution were simply desperate to control her behaviour; such places reinforced compliance and were often punitive when people showed any resistance to the will of the staff.

Jennifer is not untypical in relation to the continued use of these medications. For example, a report by University College London found that, in 2015, in a sample of 33,016 people with intellectual disability, GP records showed that more than 25% had been prescribed 'antipsychotic' medications, of whom 71% had no record of 'severe mental illness' (although we also dispute when such diagnoses are made, because of the inconsistency and poorly evidenced reasoning that was seen in Jennifer's medical reviews). Their continued use, though scandalous, still has the surface semblance of respectability, because of public respect for the medical profession, whom they consider having a strong scientific basis for their work.

"Antipsychotic drugs are designed to treat severe mental illnesses such as schizophrenia. There is very little evidence that they help to address behavioural problems not due to mental illness in people with intellectual disability."

University College London website, 2 September 2015

The large institutions have gone, but chemical control that developed in these places is alive and well in community settings that are just as medicalised as any countryside hospital.

It retains its rationale and its political power through community psychiatry, nurses sympathetic to medical models of mental illness, senior NHS professionals with these professional backgrounds, and the drug companies that create – if not conflicts of interest – then continued conflicts of ideas. Since people with severe intellectual disability have less of a voice than other patient groups, their plight is largely unheard.

No one actually showed Jennifer any love, except for Camilla. Intensive Interaction practitioners do not describe it as a form of love, but they consider the intimacy, responsiveness and gentleness of that approach to be at its centre.

"Intensive Interaction is not something we do to our partners but something we share with them, listening and responding to each other… We are looking for dialogue rather than monologue."

Caldwell & Horwood, 2008

Camilla commented about Jennifer:

> *"So much time is spent arguing about this disorder and that disorder, but no one simply spends time with Jennifer, following her lead. When she finally smiles at you, when you seem to have that moment of understanding, and she holds your hand, and clings that little bit tighter when it's time to leave... that is really being with her, that is the work I do. It is really not complicated; she just needs to feel you are present and attending."*

We would leave it there.

References

Beail N & Warden S (1995) Sexual abuse of adults with learning disabilities. *Journal of Intellectual Disability Research* **39** (5) 382-387.

Caldwell P & Horwood J (2008) *Using Intensive Interaction and Sensory Integration*. London: Jessica Kinglsey Publishers.

Moncrieff J (2009) A critique of the Dopamine Hypothesis of Schizophrenia and Psychosis. *Harvard Review of Psychiatry* **17** (3) 214-225.

Sappok T, Zepperitz S & Hudson M (2021) *Meeting Emotional Needs in Intellectual Disability.* London: Hogrefe.

Chapter 17: The Team

We're flagging

A community mental health team meets once a week in a 'flagging up' meeting. This meeting is intended to 'flag' cases where a person's complex needs might cause their current situation to collapse, so as to prevent this where possible.

The loss of dedicated professionals to do crisis work linked to the 'flagging', arguments about responsibilities and roles, the avoidance of uncomfortable interventions, a lack of specialist knowledge, over-responsibility for 'saving' clients, and a failure to define the terms of reference within the meeting, all contributed to an ailing service which could not address the deep attachment issues of the clients discussed.

Instead, the team began to resemble what Wilfred Bion (1961) described as a 'Basic Assumption Group', where the focus of the team's work was unclear, and in its place there emerged a tendency for the group to seek comfort (pleasure) instead of focusing on its primary task (helping people in pain). This would occur via (a) attacking the leadership as being impotent, focused on the irrelevant, or self-interested, (b) thinly veiled conflicts of ideas that contained elements of professional envy, and (c) powerful sub-groups proposing messianic change (a vague promise of a wonderful, resolved tomorrow) that would fail to appear, though was constantly discussed. An attempt to improve this by way of consultation is discussed.

It sometimes occurs that, by engaging with childhood adversity, trauma and attachment and presenting this work, individuals in other parts of our organisation or beyond will have an interest sparked. Often, this individual will be troubled, perhaps in the form of emotions that are not congruent with their outward success in their place of work. The feeling that 'something is missing' can be hard to articulate, and harder still to identify what this something is. Not to seem grandiose, but sometimes we were approached by people working in our own and other organisations to help them identify confused or frustrated feelings in their team, often when they had tried to help people with mild or borderline intellectual disability without success. This is not unlike someone who expects to be welcomed when they are confused or distressed; it is a sign of someone seeking a secure base/safe haven, through consulting with us or asking us for a training day.

One of these approaches was from Henrietta, a senior occupational therapist in a local mental health team. Henrietta had heard about our work via a presentation to a special interest group working across the specialties of a large mental health NHS Trust (mental health, learning disability, children's mental health, community brain injury services and neurodevelopmental services). Henrietta was promoted to a leadership position in her team and had for a long time been concerned that much of what was described in Chapter 16 (Jennifer) formed a pathway that in no way considered how childhood adversity, trauma or attachment issues were both the cause, and the way forward, for very distressed and disturbed people who came to the attention of her team. As an occupational therapist, she often conducted successful work with people in relation to building relationships and then some form of life beyond serious mental health crises in people's lives. But Henrietta told us that she felt that people with mental health problems were often left with serious problems and then discharged. There was great pressure to 'do something' that was an 'evidence-based intervention' but often this meant referring to a team that would not see her client (such as for a short course of cognitive behaviour therapy, or to a 'high threshold' longer-term therapy service, who would reject referrals that were not the 'type' of patient they felt confident in helping). At the same time, she was expected to discharge people from her own service once her own very practical and helpful work was finished. Often, this led people in obvious need of further support to face complete discharge from the Trust, which actually led in many cases with serious self-harm or even suicide, because of the implied rejection.

Not surprisingly, Henrietta was interested to hear that we sought to never discharge our clients before they felt ready themselves, and that we attended to the problems involved by trying to find caring arrangements that would feel like secure attachment caregiving.

But what was the best way of bringing our approach to Henrietta's team? She told us about a weekly meeting that was intended to prevent admissions to hospital, based on the imperfect idea that 'care in the community' is somehow healthier. Living in a hospital is now considered an evil, in sharp contrast to the post-WWII period, when institutional care for people with intellectual disabilities and people experiencing psychosis or severe depression was entirely normal. Now, even staying longer than necessary 'to treat disorder' is seen as bad practice, although it happens a lot, and at the time of writing this book, there were several thousand people[24] with intellectual disabilities still living in hospital, despite multiple policy documents and government-endorsed papers stating that these environments are inappropriate.

We negotiated from a deliberate position of naiveté, and asked Henrietta if it would be acceptable to their team for us to attend a series of their 'flagging up' meetings. These were held at the height of the COVID outbreak, and so they were held online. We joined a meeting of between ten and 20 personnel each Thursday morning for a period of ten weeks. In the first of these, we were simply added with no introductions, and with no explanation for our presence (in fairness, an email had been sent out the week before).

The meetings were, given the risks discussed, surprisingly 'flat', with a notable lack of alarm. Each week about a dozen people were discussed. To be added to the agenda of the meeting, the person had to have either threatened suicide in a credible way, neglected themselves very seriously, or been referred in by the police or psychiatric liaison services based in the local emergency department. The team leader would say, "So the next one is [client name]. Does anyone have an update?" Sometimes, an awkward silence would follow; nothing had been done, and no one was held responsible for making regular contact with the person.

In most cases, a member of the team who had the person on their caseload would give an update consisting of their clinical actions. There were instances where these were well-thought-out interventions based on theories that have a lot of currency. For example, a person who presented to A&E with an overdose was offered several sessions with a nurse to discuss ways of discharging frustration that are less dangerous, such as using a 'stress bucket'[25]. However, such interventions were never considered in term of the state of scientific evidence, rather, if someone

24 On 12th February 2023, there were just over 2,000 people with learning disabilities in England being held as in-patients on mental health wards (source: autism.org.uk).

25 The person noticing things that they find stressful, such as arguments with family, worries about finances, lack of sleep etc. then judges if their 'bucket' is getting full or not. When it is, one imagines putting the bucket down and then doing things that reduce the stress, such as 'doing something I enjoy', 'performing a relaxation technique', 'making a healthy meal' or 'talking to a friend'.

was trained in the model, then that model it was[26]. We noted that this was a general problem in the multidisciplinary team – practitioners were loyal to their own model, and indeed sometimes were 'badged' as model advocates such as 'Positive behaviour support practitioner', 'Well-being practitioner', 'cognitive behavioural therapist', or, less commonly, 'psychodynamic counsellor'.

However, the *standard update* in the meeting was generally something that lacked any theory or research basis, approximating, "I went and saw the person today. They/their staff said it was a good/bad week". A 'good week' referred to an absence of personal crises, not presenting to urgent care or crisis services, and was thus defined by an absence of negatives (rather than the presence of the fulfilling aspects of life). A 'bad week' would be reported as any attempt at self-harm, harm to others, threats or desperate acts. We noted that the people were described in terms of their behaviour, and more specifically, the *risks associated with their actions*. Risk assessment, which is pretty much the one skill shared by all mental health professionals, is the common language.

The standard update was often followed by the question as to whether the person was 'compliant with treatment' (usually medication) – what we call *compliant self-calming*. For example, the main intervention of the team was the use of depot injections of strong psychoactive substances intended to dampen hallucinations and/or delusions. This was tinged with a feeling that the person was not being a 'good patient' and in some way by not complying, the 'consequences' of not complying with the treatment plan, or respecting 'boundaries', should teach them to behave more as expected. This would emerge in comments about the person, despite their disability or illness, having 'capacity', and therefore being entirely responsible for acting in ways that are criminal, wasteful of public resources, or otherwise socially 'abnormal'. If they suffered, it was somehow deserved. We found two phenomena that would be denied here – first was the obvious need to be with others in order to calm, which was a concept the team avoided assiduously (perhaps because they feared being overwhelmed by the person's need for care or their trauma); and second, that what the patients were asking for was psychological, not chemical.

26 A scientific study of high quality, known as a 'randomised controlled trial' of a version of the stress bucket (the ReZone Self-management system) was carried out by Edridge *et al* (2020). They found that the technique did not enhance outcomes for a range of difficulties in young people (emotional difficulties, empowerment, well-being, or quality of life).

"I don't want things. I just want your time."

Roger Wilczek, expert by experience

We also noted that roles were not clearly defined, despite the development of 'care pathways'. We called this *role ambivalence*. Nurses, in particular, would often voice discomfort at being involved in a case or being required to do the standard update. Sometimes, between meetings, a professional would decide that they no longer had a role and discharge the case without consulting others involved. We found it difficult to ascertain the exact roles of the nursing team, especially with regard to psychological care. They seemed on stronger ground with the psychiatry team, with whom they would have a clear supporting role, with regard to medication, temporary holding powers in a crisis, etc. Psychologists, therapists, occupational therapists and others had fuzzier boundaries. For example, should a nurse attempt an intervention based on cognitive behaviour therapy? Sometimes this appeared to occur; at other times it was vociferously avoided as 'not within my role'. Conflict would appear between nurses and other professionals, and even between nurses, as to what they should offer. It was as though some felt betrayed by colleagues who were 'doing other people's jobs for them', or even 'teacher's pets'. However, it is important to say that nurses were not the only team members who voiced role ambivalence. Some professionals, for example, psychologists, often felt that they were being given cases without a clear care pathway in order that others would feel the relief of handing the case (and its inherent anxiety) over.

Role ambivalence was strongly related to another phenomenon, which we called *primary task avoidance*. The team's primary task was to provide assessments and interventions that would improve a person's life using evidence-based methods. The methods that are truly evidence-based for a mental health service – such as skilled counselling, psychotherapy, behavioural activation, systematic desensitisation, family therapy and attachment-based interventions – were rarely sought out, either in terms of referrals to and with the service, or by professionals seeking training. Instead, the use of psychoactive medications, brief 'coping skills' techniques, referrals to other services and unfocused home visits were prevalent. Some people were referred to psychology, but this was for 'short-term cognitive behavioural therapy' or, worst of all, 'scaffolding' (the addition of a monthly meeting by another team with the person offering the unfocused home visit). In doing these things, a semblance of activity covered the primary task avoidance. Since almost all of the people receiving the service had multiple ACEs that underpinned their particular presenting problem (severe anxiety, mood disturbance, hallucinations, delusions, self-harming by way of overdose, etc.), the primary task of the team was *essentially to help people process their trauma rather than alleviate symptoms*.

While the case can be made that this is essentially what Sigmund Freud said[27], one need not actually adhere to any psychological model of severe distress to know what overcoming trauma involves. One has to sit with someone, and without deflection or distraction, accompany them emotionally through their memories, while they create a self-validating story. This is not as simple or straightforward as it sounds in many cases, but it is still the necessary process.

Figure 17.1: The pan-theoretical process of overcoming trauma

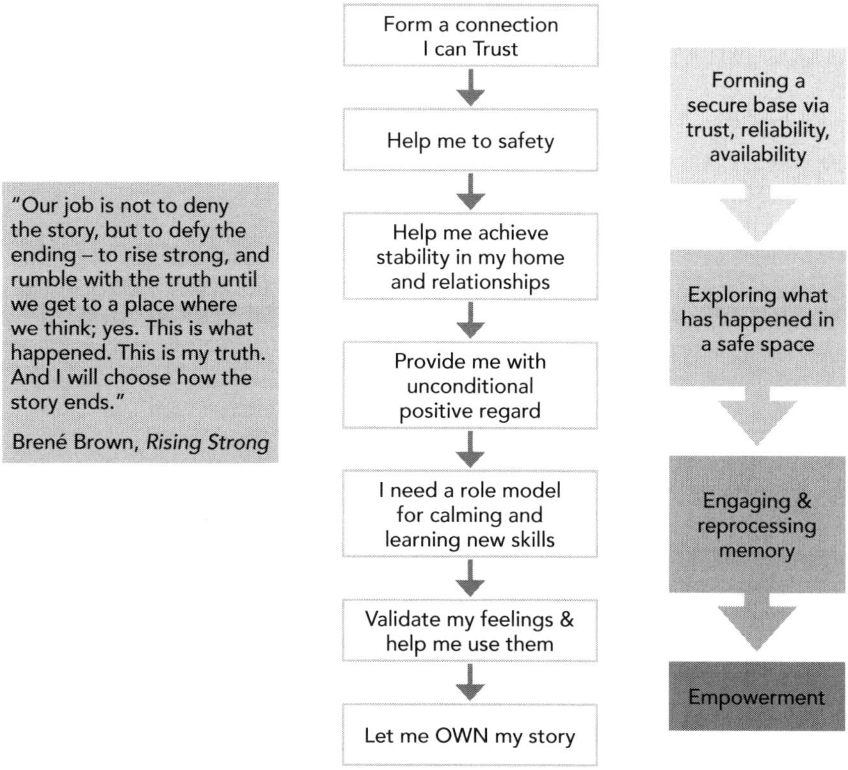

27 Among many apt comments, Freud wrote that "unexpressed emotions will never die. They are buried alive and will come forth later in uglier ways". In Freud S (1915) *Introductory Lectures in Psycho-analysis*. London: Hogarth Press.

Since sitting with someone who is deeply wounded – and trauma involves recovering from a wound – is very painful, it is very common for people to try to avoid this pain. However, alleviating deep emotional pain is very difficult and takes time – as long as it takes. Services that stipulate only a small number of sessions are by necessity limiting the effect they can have on trauma. Since we are suggesting that this can only happen via the establishment of a secure attachment to the helping person, it cannot be done by self-help or by simply following written instructions. Moreover, techniques such as snapping elastic bands on wrists or mindfulness exercises etc. can only have an effect where there is sufficient trust in the self. This self-trust can only be present in those people who have had strong childhood building blocks (their parents engaged in sufficient secure caregiving attachment behaviours).

Other processes seemed to reflect a kind of *them and us* phenomenon. For example, the local authority, it was felt, were not pulling their weight, finding the right accommodation, or moving quickly enough to support people. They were also perceived as wanting people to remain in healthcare settings as this meant that they did not have to pay for the care. Health professionals could therefore sit in the relatively comfortable position of being able to blame others for a person's predicament. Such relief is only temporary, though, as we noted that, when there were actual conversations with the local authority, they had indeed worked as hard as possible with the cases, done their assessments in a timely way, and were themselves bound by factors outside of their control. They were not 'them' at all.

One way of understanding a group dynamic is to think of an organisation as having anxiety in the same way as an organism (e.g., a person) might have anxiety. This *organisational anxiety* is to some extent built from the individual anxieties of healthcare professionals, the appropriate anxiety they should feel in relation to their healthcare tasks, and the stresses and supports of working in an organisation that tries to help people who are highly distressed. Professionals may think, "Have I done everything I should have?", or "I wonder if other professionals should be doing more?" Less consciously, they may be worried about being blamed, shamed, or even professionally destroyed by some form of failure in one's duty. When a person dies in a healthcare setting, there is an investigation and some form of 'lessons learned', an inquest, and scrutiny of what help they received or did not receive. Understandably, professionals ask questions of themselves, but it is unrealistic to expect that being involved in such processes will not happen throughout an entire career in mental health services. Some people will die, and others will not have good outcomes.

The great fear, that was almost impossible to acknowledge, was that some aspects of disability, the person's life before they came to the notice of the team, and their social and economic position, could not be altered greatly. At a fundamental level, professionals choose their careers to find a role that they find satisfying. This has been long known.

> "*We know that doctors and nurses undertake the work of alleviating suffering because of deep personal reasons… we also know that if human needs are not satisfied, they tend to become more passionate, to be reinforced by aggression, and then to deteriorate in maturity, with sadism invading the situation, together with its concomitants of anxiety, guilt, depression and compulsive reparative wishes, until ultimate despair can ensue.*"
>
> TF Main, *The Ailment*, 1957

These phenomena remind us of Malan'ss ***triangle of conflict***, which is a psychodynamic representation of how difficult feelings can be avoided either in an individual or in a group of people. Anxiety rises, perhaps due to guilt caused by a team not quite knowing how to soothe a person in extreme distress, due to unprocessed trauma (which is a strong basis for severe and enduring distress, often called 'mental illness').

Figure 17.2: Relationship of anxiety about complex cases to group defences and the associated feelings that are avoided (derived from Malan's Triangle of Conflict[28])

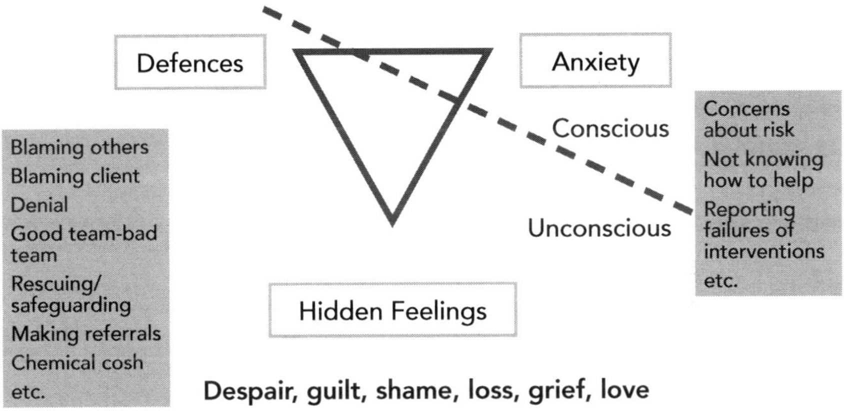

We were also aware that our growing sense of the prevalence, multiplicity and pervasiveness of the traumas and poor attachment histories of our own patients had started to wear on us. We were suffering vicarious moral injury, through the sheer injustice of unacknowledged trauma in the people we worked with, which can be seen throughout this book. Working with Henrietta's team reminded us that this is common in healthcare teams who have not properly defined their roles and the main work of their service, and they therefore become distracted by internal conflict and conflict with other groups and organisations. It was therefore important for us to seek our own support in order to prevent us attacking, rescuing, rubbishing or despairing about our colleagues.

Wilfred Bion's seminal work on group behaviour is well summarised for healthcare teams by Jon Stokes (1994). The paper *Problems in Multidisciplinary Teams* could almost have described word for word what was happening to Henrietta's service. Stokes describes, with tragi-comic accuracy, a community team meeting degenerating into debates about the relative merits of different types of chair, which room to hold the meeting in, and whether the meeting was 'good' or 'bad'. Stokes noted that this was usually to avoid conflict between members.

28 The Malan Triangles, comprising the triangle of conflict and the triangle of persons, were developed in 1979 by David Malan as a way of illuminating the concept of transference in psychotherapy situations. These triangles are considered main components in some forms of psychotherapy, and are widely used in training, research, and other works. A reference is included at the end of this chapter.

Stokes applies Wilfred Bion's *Experiences in Groups* (1961) to discuss how community teams can, because of the difficulty and emotional pain of their actual commissioned work, become avoidant of this pain and instead focus on keeping everyone in the team comfortable. This is indeed very apt in mental health and learning disability teams, where work can be hard to define and roles quite fuzzy. Three processes can occur – Basic Assumption Leadership, 'fight or flight', or Basic Assumption Pairing. These are 'basic assumptions' because they are unconscious fall-backs to our need for others to care for us, and for us to be the focus of a group – to have our needs met as if we were emotionally dependent children.

Basic Assumption Leadership

All leadership roles, such as community team managers, engage in a mix of Basic Assumption Leadership (BAL) and Primary Task Leadership (PTL). It is possible to tell if one or the other is dominating because when teams are focused on their primary task, they find it relatively easy to describe the function of their team. This is easier with some briefs than with others. For example, a team with generic roles will find that PTL is not easy to define because teams are often formed because of legacy roles (as with the closure of long-stay hospitals requiring the redeployment of many nurses, nursing assistants, psychiatrists, etc.) or because the services are provided in the community. This can make it difficult for a team to articulate its function. In the case of a breast screening unit, the role is relatively simple: to screen a given population at risk of breast cancer, detect potentially abnormal results, and forward these to specialists for further investigation and intervention as necessary. In a mental health team, there are multiple roles that are loosely focused on preventing and reducing mental distress in its more extreme forms, but the task is varied[29]. Some are focused on risk assessment, some on drug treatments, some on psychological interventions, some on occupational therapy interventions, some on admission to hospital and discharge, etc. Care Co-ordination is intended to prevent the various professionals from simply doing their own thing, but this can become a process which feels automatic and does not

29 This is even more true in learning disability teams, where the team is named *for the condition of having a learning disability*, as though it was something that might be cured. Not only are roles largely non-overlapping (e.g. physiotherapy vs psychiatry vs dietetics), but often referrals are made to assess the learning disability without any obvious need for clinical intervention. Such teams often struggle to say in a single sentence what their team does, which makes defining and focusing on a Primary Task very difficult.

imply the urgent necessity for improvement in the condition of the person referred to the service.

Process goals, so often how teams are evaluated (so many assessments will be completed, a percentage of risk assessments will be completed, the person's ethnicity or employment status will be recorded, etc.) are a large part of the problem. Effective teams should be focused on outcomes, not processes, with process goals designed to improve the efficient throughput of cases to achieve these outcomes. An effective team can tell you what they want to achieve in a single sentence – or even a short phrase. An example might be 'to measurably improve quality of life for our clients'. In a short phrase, this statement implies an outcome that is scientifically measurable, and if improvement has not happened over a given time period, the team will be sharply redirected to its function.

Sadly, we would contend that most community teams are not accountable in this way. They rarely use nationally benchmarked outcome tools, and improvement is ascertained as often as not by the subjective opinion of the professional involved. Teams are increasingly focused on doing healthcare processes quickly, notably in the form of eliminating the infamous *waiting list* (the time taken from referral to being seen). A team can be deemed to be successful when it sees clients quickly and discharges them promptly, having done as short an intervention as possible. Readers will note our problem with such 'light touch' teams and, without serious research into their outcomes, they will continue to appear to be doing a good job, as they 'see lots of people quite quickly'[30].

When BAL dominates, the operational leader of the team, typically a team manager, is often a popular person who is known to help others. They are experienced as someone who should lead the group (team) and members feel comfortable and not exposed to emotional pain or other discomfort. To the extent that they provide this help, they are loved and considered supportive, but the team member is free to be completely ineffective in their role, which they may not even be able to define clearly. Job descriptions are

30 But are such services any help, really? In 2014-15, there were nearly 1.3 million referrals to the Improved Access to Psychological Therapies (IAPT) service in England. Of these, 815,665 (63%) entered treatment, of whom only 37% (about 300,000) completed the sessions. However, only 180,300 were found to have 'reliable recovery' on standardised measures of 'anxiety' and 'depression'. Even if we accept the criteria for success, which are a questionably low-bar, this represents only about 14% of the people referred. It could be argued that the huge diversion of resources to IAPT, based as it was on limited evidence presented by advocates of the cognitive-behaviour therapy movement, and the economist Richard Layard, has been a failure in both process (cannot get most people through the therapy) and outcome (only 14% of people referred achieving reduced anxiety and depression scores).

no help, being written in vague process-based language, e.g. 'the post-holder will provide evidence-based interventions to address a wide range of clinical problems that are seen by the community mental health team'. These documents tend to neither specify the role particularly, nor to provide clear, measurable outcomes by which accountability will be determined[31].

Henrietta's team was led by Johan, a man in his mid-60s approaching retirement. Johan has worked for most of his career as a physiotherapist, largely working independently and with a large caseload and high work rate (a high number of appointments per working day). Johan was popular with the organisation's management as he was so busy and the model of a hard worker, who was seemingly inexhaustible. Most of his day was taken up with management supervisions, partly due to the flat management structure of the team. However, he was also asked for a lot of clinical advice, which he freely gave but which was beyond his qualifications and expertise. The office was open plan, and Johan would always sit with the group, waiting for professionals to come and go from their appointments and home visits, to welcome them, make tea and offer constant support. He was seen as unthreatening but also feckless and incompetent. Several members of staff were absent with stress-related conditions, citing problems with the working relationship with Johan as at least part of the reason for being off. Johan could be contacted out of office hours. He was available for calls from the crisis team as well as the community team.

Johan's *self-appointed impossible task*, to make everyone in the team feel loved, was at the expense of never addressing conflicts between team members, that were quite serious in nature. Some influential team members were clearly projecting feelings of depression within the team, such as by loudly saying "Oh, I can't be bothered today" in the office or asking about each other's private lives in unwanted ways, or concerns being expressed about team members not pulling their weight. Other conflicts included near-open contempt for each other's skill sets, the 'not my job' phenomenon, and resistance to referrals that went far beyond the criteria for entry into the team for help.

---

31 The introduction of outcome measures can be fiercely resisted, on apparent 'scientific' grounds, or 'unfairness' such as some team members seeing more 'complex' cases than others, but this is really because it would expose the team members' focus on their own comfort and the need for the leader to protect them. It is entirely possible that a negative evaluation of a person's clinical interventions can be rationalised as resulting from 'bullying' by the leader, resulting in a long period of stress-related sickness, and the invocation of the bullying & harassment and grievance policies of the organisation. It is often very difficult to determine if a staff member is actually being harassed or is avoiding scrutiny of their performance; and of course, these are not mutually exclusive possibilities.

Some team members responded to the lack of resolution by openly or covertly despising Johan or displacing this onto other staff. Some made fun of him as a "cuddly father figure" who "couldn't discipline a puppy". Meanwhile, Johan had to attend meetings with more senior managers, who considered him to be the opposite – rude but achieving good outcomes for clients (which were in fact process goals, which had nothing to do with outcome). For example, he was commended for the short waiting times in the service.

Feedback to us from other staff included widely varying views of Johan. They could not all be true as they were completely opposing ideas. However, they did broadly paint a picture of a manager who wanted to keep everyone happy, but who rarely addressed the real needs of the client group. Patient experience surveys of the team were actually quite negative (with some very positive exceptions) and suggested that the team were very focused on doing as little work with clients as possible before 'stepping them down' to primary care, and that it was normal for a team member who worked for more than a few weeks with the clients to be considered indulgent and weak, if not actually incompetent (as good interventions are short, skills-based and effective).

Thinking more about the conflicts between team members, the basic assumption process of *Fight or Flight* needs to be explained. Clinicians will be aware that not everyone in their organisation likes them as much as others do. This natural variation is exaggerated by the powerful emotions introduced by the casework.

Conflicted role can then arise because of unconscious envies, rivalries, and competing models. These include the role of *rescuer*, where the professional fantasises, and perhaps acts, as though they will save the situation or the person. This is often based on the actual or presumed transgression of an important principle, such as raising concerns about the person being denied access to a service, or another form of accusing others of 'withholding'. One example of this is a client who was repeatedly referred for a particular psychological therapy which their family doctor believed to match the person's condition. Prior assessments had indicated that the person lacked motivation to change their actions and opinions, and instead firmly believed that other people were to blame for their situation. To the extent that this was partially true (they had indeed been maltreated in the past), the helpful line of action was to seek help in the advocacy process for seeking justice. However, this required action from the client themselves, rather than the professional. The referring doctor became somewhat discredited among colleagues as too 'personally involved' with the client. The 'super-clinician' who 'goes the extra mile' can be prone to moving beyond the boundaries of their professional role, which can eventually lead to burn-out, depression and hopelessness.

On the other side of this dynamic, it is rather easy to fall into the *victim* role. In the above example, the imagined 'withholding' therapist felt attacked and denigrated. Rather than holding onto these feelings and processing them as part of understanding how the named client may be acting out, it can be very tempting simply to put up a stalwart defence of one's position. This can lead to terse letters between professionals who openly disagree and / or align or stand against the person's demands. Interestingly, such disagreements rarely flare into open conflict with formal meetings and proceedings. It is much more likely in our experience that the professionals avoid each other and / or avoid talking about the issue, and in a sense the person simply re-enacts their internalised family (in this case, that parents were experienced as uncaring and unavailable) within the 'family' of the clinical service.

The third point of this dysfunctional triad is the *persecutor* role. Less easy to gain insight into (for who wants to be seen as persecutory?), this often occurs when something more sadistic and vengeful enters the situation, and a feeling of "rooting out the bad apples" takes over. Typically, this is the unpopular manager who finally wants to grasp the nettle to end a conflict, perhaps on the back of poor performance in a worker, or to overcome obstacles to organisational change. It can also occur easily when victims and rescuers attack others in the defence of their position. Unwittingly, they have become the persecutor[32].

As alluded to in the above example, both Stokes (1994) and Bion (1961) point out that in *Fight or Flight*, it is important that the conflict is known about but not resolved. The antagonists do not contact each other and are unlikely to collaborate closely, with any unavoidable meetings being frosty and with conflicts unsaid. Voluntary projects are never joined by both parties spontaneously. They circle each other, never meeting, ready to attack or run, but rarely engaging directly in an argument. They may gather followers whom they convince, with varying levels of subtlety, that the other

32 The triad above has been named the *drama triangle* by Karpman (1968) which he developed as a description of destructive interactions. It is a powerful model of problematic relations in its own right, based in the Transactional Analysis school of psychotherapy.

person is 'bad'. The organisation is much more likely to move one or both parties to a new department rather than sit down with them to resolve any differences. Such conflicts successfully distract the team from the failure to complete the primary task, which is what is truly being avoided.

In the team that Henrietta invited us to support, Johan confided that he was extremely worried about the relationship between Henrietta and Jonathan, a social worker. They often disagreed vehemently about their cases. Henrietta was given to a basically medical model of psychological distress. She firmly believed that the unmet need for clear medical diagnosis was depriving people of the right drug-based treatments that would allow them relief from their distress and support them to engage more in work, leisure and social activities. While there may be difficulties with side effects and becoming dependent on medication, these were secondary to the primary benefit of medication, according to Henrietta. She pointed to studies showing large reductions in medical symptoms in studies of people with 'schizophrenia', 'major depression' and 'bipolar disorder' following the administration of powerful drugs. She was 'standing by science'.

Jonathan believed strongly that most of a person's mental health problems were socially determined: unemployment, poor-quality housing, negative attitudes from 'neurotypical people', benefit cuts and, ultimately, conservative political philosophy. He believed that the studies Henrietta talked about were flawed, with publication bias[33], questionable control groups[34], and unreliable diagnoses[35]. He also felt that he was standing by science, but science with a proper critique.

When we raised the conflict of ideas in our consultation, the argument did come out into the open. Jonathan said that he found it professionally and personally difficult even to hear the words that Henrietta used, as he perceived words like 'schizophrenic' to be profoundly oppressive – a label that would instantly stigmatise a person and cause them to lose

33 Publication bias refers to a tendency of a body with vested interests (e.g. pharmaceuticals companies) to publish only those studies which show that their treatments work.

34 Many groups of patients used to compare the effects of drugs in people given a new drug during a trial are described as having 'treatment as usual' (TAU), but they are often actually recently withdrawn from a drug. Many have argued that this is an unfair comparison because these 'control groups' are actually people in cold turkey, and not being treated with an alternative drug.

35 It is well known that psychiatric diagnoses are not made reliably enough (i.e., different professionals will diagnose different conditions with the same information) and this questions the very validity of the diagnoses. Given that a psychiatric diagnosis has a powerful effect on a person's life, this continues to be concerning.

social opportunities, to be considered a bad bet for employers, and to be stuck on powerful medications that did not, over the long term, serve to help them. Jonathan was also very critical of the team's focus – driven by considerable anxiety – on making sure depot injections were given at the right time, to prevent a person becoming very distressed, or, as several team members called it, 'ill'. It was, however, relatively easy to discuss the conceptual disagreements between Henrietta and Jonathan. Other team members were very emollient, and Johan went out of his way to allow 'different views', and to have separate meetings where he seemed to agree with both parties, even when their beliefs about a case would take it in starkly different directions. In writing, Jonathan openly opposed several diagnostic assessments by Henrietta and other psychiatrists, which they considered insulting at a personal level, and implying not only that they were incompetent at applied science, but actually engaged in the oppression of people at vulnerable times in their lives, selling snake oil to anaesthetise them from their maltreatment or their social conditions. It was society that was mad, not the patients[36].

We noted that in both approaches it was not necessary to meet with clients very much. Henrietta would see clients for an initial assessment and then do a clinic review many months later, even up to six months unless there was a sharp increase in concern. Jonathan would assess and then, mostly, make recommendations to the local authority to increase money or care arrangements for the person. It was clear that both did have some worry that their work was not actually particularly effective, and their largely academic disagreements, which were rarely face to face, were never resolved. Both were relatively comfortable in their positions, even when their differing views caused confusion in patients who would often have to make a choice as to whom they wanted to believe. Many patients would see both almost as a parallel process; while there was thinly veiled hostility communicated to patients in subtle and not-so-subtle ways, they rarely stopped their medication on the basis of what Jonathan said, nor did they stop the social interventions that Jonathan would instigate. With Johan's help, the team muddled through with a mixture of avoidance, jokes about the conflict, and denial. This resulted in Henrietta and Jonathan largely circling each other warily, but never engaging in the painful dialectic that would have started to resolve their disagreement. Both had a lot to lose; their very understanding, their story about why

36 This view was actually arrived at in the 1960s by RD Laing, who considered 'madness' a sane response to impossible psychological dilemmas that we can find ourselves in.

people become chronically and severely distressed. At a deeper level, we sensed that Henrietta and Jonathan were both attracted to interaction with each other, as each represented what their families had lacked; for Henrietta, family 'mental illnesses' had gone unchecked for many years, and in a moment of irritation with Jonathan, she disclosed this in a professional meeting, hence her "passion for psychiatry". Jonathan was less disposed to explanation in this way, but it was well known 'through the grapevine' that Jonathan had come from an area of economic deprivation and was equally passionate about the need to emancipate the country from poverty. His work was essentially a mission to end the mental illness model and replace it with a model of economic equality, that would remove the reasons for the mental illness narrative.

When Jonathan announced his retirement, Henrietta was relieved. This reduced the conflict but also unbalanced the team towards a traditional medical model of mental illness. Other team members, who had partly or wholly agreed with Jonathan, expressed that they felt that patients were seen as malfunctioning machinery, and that the new approach lacked any understanding of the social reasons for mental health diagnoses. We fed back that something was lost here; the team's assumptions became too certain, and the understanding of patients' lives too simplistic, ahistorical, and biological. Nevertheless, the simplification of roles, particularly for community nurses, seemed to offer some relief to them – they no longer feared weekly meetings. Johan was particularly pleased; there was great joy and gratitude shown to Jonathan during his final months, but we felt that this was as much about their pleasure in him going as about celebrating his contribution. All of the conflict, though it seemed to be about 'right and wrong', with both sides feeling they were in the right, failed to think, ever, about how this acting-out affected the patients. It was like a family in which the parents hated each other but refused to split up, leading to neglect of their charges. Writing righteous emails was preferred to visiting the patients, and the team became focused on the relationship between Jonathan and Henrietta, rather than the need for patients to reprocess a traumatic past.

The *Basic Assumption Pairing* (BaP) also involves a strong emotional dynamic that diverts from the need for potentially uncomfortable working that would improve actual outcomes. Typically, pairs of professionals embark on an important-soundingproject that is only loosely related to outcome, often an ethical principle (such as equality of access to a service) or an organisational process which is seen as inefficient or unsatisfactory. In Henrietta's service, two senior professionals, George and Lucy, were appointed as organisation-wide consultants to develop a new protocol to reduce waiting times to less than four weeks from referral to first appointment. They embarked on a long period of consultation, asking for staff to complete a survey about current practices, and then meeting several times each week to discuss the results. The resulting report, which took almost two years to produce, was much anticipated by managers as an important answer to an irksome requirement for the service to 'do something like an assessment' within about a month of referral.

However, the report caused a huge upset in the team when it arrived. Far from being experienced as a welcome solution, team members felt like they had been labelled as lazy, if not completely feckless. Some meetings to introduce the new policy became very heated, with staff being upset about the report to the point where it seemed like a personal attack; while in other meetings, the staff refused to comment or ask questions, which led to awkward silences and a failure to engage with the policy. Due to the extreme responses of some staff, and poor general engagement, the policy was watered down with a long implementation time of a further two years and a vague commitment that George and Lucy would be available to discuss the policy with any staff who contacted them. None did. Within the 'probationary' period, both George and Lucy obtained new promotions and left the organisation. No one else seemed to pick up the policy, and waiting times continued to be both an annoyance to the managers and a consistent feature of the patient experience. Currently, no one even talks about the project, which has been quietly 'shelved', but not in a conscious way – everyone involved who still works there seems incapable of remembering it as a failure.

It has been noted that such pairings are akin, in some ways, to adult sexual relationships. There may be jokes about being 'work partners', or jealous jibes implying that they more than work together. The couple need not consciously experience anything sexual, nor show any behaviour towards each other that is considered inappropriate, but that does not stop the tongues from wagging. In psychoanalytic theory, this is entirely expected; indeed, a kind of repressed desire for each other is a (the) source of the drive for the Basic Assumption Pair to work together. They are indeed *sublimated* work spouses; there will be no physical contact, but they are emotionally connected. It is worth saying that, when paired with a focus on the real work – the primary task – (George and Lucy did not have caseloads while working on the project), the unsaid sexual chemistry can be powerfully productive. The resonance with the idea of Messiah will also not be lost on many readers – a man and a woman promise that with the coming of their 'baby' (a project is often referred to as 'our baby'), things will be better, more secure; we will be more deserving of approval. The Basic Assumption Pairing is, above all, a fantasy. There will be no bright new tomorrow, there will only be a continual offering of more painful graft, or more avoidance of this graft, through basic assumption processes and other defences.

The reality of staffing in Henrietta's team belied just how much the team had turned away from its actual work, which one could argue to be supporting people to reprocess their childhood and recent traumas. Some might argue that such teams should only do enough to help people function in their family life and jobs, but we know that longer and psychologically deeper interventions can have better outcomes (Knekt *et al*, 2008). Staff were sometimes redeployed (three psychologists, two nurses, six occupational therapists, two healthcare assistants), and other staff left or retired, with the posts being deleted to save money (four full-time posts). Some professions had real difficulties with recruiting even one member of a core profession, so that the consultant psychiatrist was shared across this team and two others, and prescribing was shared with nurses who had done a prescribing course in order to address this[37] (prescribing without the anatomy and physiology training of medical personnel). Still others found their roles changed or limited in ways that disallowed them from addressing the primary task; some were diverted into projects, like patient satisfaction surveys, an initiative to get all clients reviewed by their GPs on an annual basis to prevent internal bodily damage from the use of lithium, or other procedural tasks that had no effect on the person's well-being.

Intervention

Our intervention was made tentatively and in the context of experiencing silence, which we considered potentially hostile or fearful. After attending

37 This was deeply concerning to the organisation's psychiatrists, who were very uneasy about the safety of nurse prescribing and the supervision of their work. It is unclear if this was justified or whether it was 'Fight or Flight' because the disagreement was never discussed and processed between the two people who were most at loggerheads about it. It just 'hung around', creating an unresolved feeling that was perceived as unsafe.

four 'Flaggings', we asked if we could give some feedback. We did this in the form of a statement which was then open to questions and comments.

Our statement at Flagging #5 was as follows:

> This team is made up of compassionate and dedicated people who really want to ensure that people with severe mental health problems and additional disabilities get better. It is certainly reassuring when there is success. The team might want to consider if there is a form of words that would capture this success in a way that encapsulates the work of everyone; for example, 'to improve a person's quality of life', or 'reducing distress and confusion for people in adversity'. These 'main outcomes' should be easily quantified at the level of human feedback, at the level of the clinical outcome scale, and at the level of aggregated outcomes or even audit and research.
>
> We do not suggest that you define your core team outcomes (and therefore your joint mission) to reduce the worries experienced by higher members of your organisation, nor to meet arbitrary targets. We want you all to be able to articulate what we call the team's *primary task*. A primary task should be defined which encompasses everything that you do, in terms of the outcome achieved. It could be as simple as 'empowerment' or 'improving quality of life', but it must be measurable at all levels and regularly reviewed. If any team does not do this, it begins to gravitate towards comfort and coasting, and avoids work that is uncomfortable or painful. When the shared primary task is not clear, we can find ourselves doing and saying things that may not be consistent with this outcome, or simply try to achieve targets for their own sake. A target culture, as opposed to an outcome culture, is demoralising and doesn't foster positive relationships with each other. The best that one can expect in a target culture is to be told that you have been satisfactorily compliant this month, as though you are schoolchildren being praised by teaching staff.
>
> There is clearly some basic conflict about the underlying philosophies at work in this team. Some people believe that they are treating medical illnesses, that may have mixed biological, social and familial causes, but can be treated with drug treatments that alter brain chemistry. This has clear currency in a trust that defines itself as a Mental Health Trust, since the metaphor of 'mental health' idea

implies 'mental illness'. Some team members do not believe in mental illness in the way it has been described for about 70 years. They have allied themselves to models that are currently quite innovative, which could be characterised as 'distress as unexpressed trauma'. This leads to an honest and principled debate about whether the patients served are hurt or harmed by our underlying working models, which also reflect our personal beliefs. One point to make about this is that it represents the struggle in the wider clinical and research communities between these models. At the coal face, however, disagreements based on fundamental differences of principle can feel very personal. Being kind folk, we do not like to hurt our colleagues and undermine their profession. Therefore, we might engage in avoidance – in our minds and in our behaviour – so that we avoid the conflict, and it is never resolved. This was called 'Fight or Flight' in the work of the psychoanalyst Wilfred Bion. This should not be confused with the widely known behavioural-physiological model of adrenaline release when we are under threat – though adrenaline may be involved. It refers instead to a kind of unresolved, unstated, but known conflict between individuals in the team.

This is not the only conflict, however. Some people are committed to efficient, relatively fast interventions, because they want as many patients to receive good, standardised care as is possible to achieve. This can push a person towards activity targets, to see as many patients as possible. But we also note that almost everyone in the team is avoiding transparent audit of their patient outcomes. This speaks to a fear – which is very human – that we may not be as good as our own personal standards demand. It is therefore easier for Johan to compliment us on how many people we see, our short waiting list, and our rate of discharge, than to ask us to check our outcomes against national benchmarks, or more deeply, for a clinical supervision group to discuss the painful difficulties of complex cases. Complexity seems reserved for this meeting, the 'Flagging' meeting.

The wry among you may have noted the double meaning of 'flagging'. We do wonder if this communicates, unconsciously, that the team 'flags' – indicates by waving a (white?) flag, but also loses impetus and potency, when cases are hard to help. A few members of the team seem aware that there is something unsatisfactory about this, and we note that these members may have on the one hand lost faith in the multidisciplinary project, preferring instead to work alone or within their profession, but who are also mostly working long-term with clients. This work may not be as focused as it could be, but on the other hand, we know from research that long-term work may be necessary for people in enduring distress. Referring to psychological treatments, the clinician and writer Adam Philips commented that this work is, 'above all, about time'. We support longer-term working and committing to a substantive relationship with clients who struggle in the longer term. However, we suggest that it would help if those who work in this way were less isolated and reached out to the wider team by attending MDT meetings more regularly, so that other team members can support them and so that others can learn the value of deeper connections to the clients.

It is possible for a group to be depressed. All groups tend to contain depressed feelings, and we probably vacillate between feeling effective and ineffective, as positive and negative information is shared about client progress. We have noted that the 'standard update' in the flagging meeting leads to more inertia in the meeting than feedback about a specific intervention where a professional has unique expertise. We suggest that this is because detailed, tangible interventions meet the primary task of improving the patient's life, whereas the standard update only offers a kind of reduction in team anxiety through staying abreast of events. When the standard update, role confusion, and unresolved conflict in the models of care are too prominent, the group will become depressed and rather hopeless about the patients.

Johan has the impossible task of keeping everyone happy when the work itself derives from deep personal losses, trauma that has led to deep shame, a cutting off or 'dissociation' from memories of these experiences, and physiological disturbances that are also commonly derived from this distress, such as severe sleep disturbances and loss of appetite. Some people even have delusions and hallucinations that could be seen as symbolising their traumatic experiences. It is impossible to gloss over how such deep psychic pain is mirrored in the helpers, and it must sometimes be expressed in conflicts between professionals. Groups can also be eviscerating of leaders who do not keep their members comfortable and free from distress, just as parents who are felt to be unfair to their children become objects of attack and ridicule. It may help to further try to understand Johan's position when we want something from him, such as new resources or when he is asked to resolve a difference of opinion. While he can certainly help in many if not most situations, he also lacks the magical ability to make the work painless. We acknowledge his powerful efforts in trying to square so many circles and ask that others be patient when conflicts arise.

The waiting list project by George and Lucy was not successful in reducing waiting times, still less in improving morale. Some group members felt attacked by the report, and this may be partly due to the factors that people felt were out of their control, such as when a clinician has to wait beyond the standard waiting time because they are waiting for someone else to complete an action. It may also be due to a real need for staff to step up and step into their workloads with more gusto, without this being a denial of previous good work, or besmirching anyone's professionalism or character. The terms of the initiative were never agreed with the group, and many team members did not see that reducing waiting times is a key area for improvement. We noted that team members rarely speak of clinical outcomes; in fact, clinical outcomes are not really defined. They are rather assumed and seen in comments by patients and their carers that they are 'fine' or 'settled'. An alternative view, of course, is that being compliant with societal norms is in fact simply glossing over our deeper need to be heard and our trials and tribulations to be understood. Patients may need to feel worse before they feel better; a breakdown may be a breakthrough; feeling sad, lost or bewildered may be a rational response to one's life circumstances. But whether one believes that reductions in symptoms or behaviours that challenge are what we are after, or simply mundane gloom in place of misery, reductions in waiting times are not in and of themselves an outcome. Functions and processes should follow our mission. They should not lead it.

We recommend three actions for your team:

1. Define what your **primary task** is as a team and consider how the processes of your team achieve this. You should define your task as an outcome and not just a process. You may need a full away day to agree this and have the session facilitated, as conflict may arise about what the team is for.

2. Ask all team members to explain the pathways of care that their patients follow, and how they meet the team's primary task. Notice, in particular, where a lack of skilled interventions is replaced by the standard update, which we see as an unhelpful defensive mechanism implying gaps in knowledge, skills and experience.
3. Since your outcomes will now be measurable, they should be measured against national benchmarks. This will reality-test if the team is doing what it should be doing.

There will be anxieties about this work, and this is normal. Working to reduce enduring distress and mental disturbance, without anxiety and uncertainty, is not likely to be effective. Discard all bureaucracy that you can within the limits of the organisation, and discuss the cases and support each other with empathy, unconditional regard, and honesty. You could use a weekly supervision group for this, but team members need to show up, both physically and emotionally. Not everyone likes to do this; some of us were discouraged from talking about our feelings as children. We expect rejection and criticism when this is done. There is no other way to stay focused on your work, however. Avoidance is the enemy, and engagement – in a trusting and supportive context – is always the way.

Feedback

There were several comments in the initial feedback about us being wily, shrewd observers. Several people mentioned that they felt rather blindsided, as they had forgotten that we were there. Johan was very ingratiating, with effusive thanks for the intervention, even though it implied that there were serious issues with the way he managed avoidance within the team. We wondered if this 'return to type' was an initial response that was almost reflexive for him, but we had hope that he would (perhaps unconsciously) move towards more painful but fruitful engagement in discussion and reflection in order to (a) harness conflict to see what ideas and practices could emerge that support the primary task, (b) allow a combination of positive and negative feedback to be given to Johan's supervisees, rather than simply trying not to upset members of staff, and (c) prevent process-based projects from becoming distractions from real service improvement.

Formal questionnaires and rating scales about this intervention were positive (e.g. a mean score of 4.7 out of 5 for unhelpful vs. helpful, where least helpful would be scored 0 and perfectly helpful would be scored 5). Yet we remain more interested in actual behavioural change within the team that would show more engagement with the primary task. Initially, the team moved towards the adoption of an outcome measure, and several were suggested, but the latest we heard was that it was found to be difficult to find a measure that was acceptable to all in the team, and this had rumbled on for several months without any real progress. One could see this as the re-emergence of Basic Assumption processes in place of primary task focus, due to the potential for discomfort in actually *choosing an outcome* and seeing how they performed to meet it. This could be personal (Johan finding it too hard to bear that he may be disliked by the staff) or due to incompatible ideas that could not be integrated (such as the medical and trauma-based models of mental distress), or due to the group making an implicit but powerful choice to stay comfortable. As with any patient of the psychotherapist, the real *work* requires pain and relinquishment of prior ideas and defences, which may simply have been too difficult for the team. However, just as a jury cannot really 'disregard' a statement made and then struck down by a judge, no matter how they are instructed to do so, named group defences are forever changed by becoming known. This 'ripple' effect can be difficult to perceive or measure, but many would say it is observed in response to unconscious processes being illuminated.

Nevertheless, the model of within-organisation-but-outside-the-team consultation using the principles introduced by Bion, and developed by Stokes, has become known as a helpful response to teams with seemingly impossible tasks[38]. It has been positively received by some key figures

38 This is not the only model that we use to conceptualise group functioning. For example, readers will have noticed features of the *Transactional Analysis* model. There is another very useful model within the psychoanalytic tradition; that of *Deep Roles*. We note that some groups actually seem to assign polarised roles that are based on early experiences of family and the roles of Mother, Father, Son and Daughter, as described by Moxnes (1999). Moxnes proposed that there are 12 'archetypal' roles that we are sucked into when we work in an organisation. Unconsciously, groups will at times of anxiety polarise these roles, so that leaders can be experienced as 'god', 'devil', 'queen', 'witch', but other team members can be a 'crown prince' or 'black sheep'. Some women may be experienced as 'princess' or 'whore'. There are also models of 'helping' roles which carry their own power in dynamics, such as the 'shaman' (wise person) or the 'slave' (who works very hard without recognition or reward). Finally, Moxnes proposes the 'hero' in a group who promises rescue, and the 'clown' who is the opposite, a pathetic 'loser'. The point of this model is to suggest that groups may function utilising cultural mythology to act as defences against the complexity and difficulty of organisational work, and by identifying someone else in a particular deep role, one does not have to attribute those imagined characteristics to oneself. For example, a worker who is worried about his or her efficacy in the role may decide that another team member is the 'clown', who is the 'loser' in the team, which lessens their conscious awareness of their own shortcomings.

See Moxnes P (1999) Deep roles: twelve primordial roles of mind and organisation. *Human Relations* **52** (11) 1427-1444.

in the organisation, and many people have voiced a beneficial – and validating – function. Healthcare teams can indeed become so distressed that they fail to complete their intended tasks, but equally they can, with the right support and intervention, come to understand the need to drop the comfortable positions and truly witness and transform the lives of those they fully mean to help.

References

Bion W (1961) *Experiences in Groups*. London: Tavistock.

Karpman S (1968) Fairy tales and script drama analysis. *Transactional Analysis Bulletin*, **26** (7) 39-43.

Malan D (1995) *Individual Psychotherapy and the Science of Psychodynamics*. Oxford: Butterworth-Heinemann.

Stokes J (1994) Problems in multidisciplinary teams: the unconscious at work. *Journal of Social Work Practice* **8** (2) 161-167.

Knekt P, Lindfors O, Laaksonen MA, Raitasalo R, Haaramo P & Järvikoski A (2008) Effectiveness of short-term and long-term psychotherapy on work ability and functional capacity; A randomized clinical trial on depressive and anxiety disorders. *Journal of Affective Disorders*, **107** (1-3) 95-106.

Chapter 18: What the science says

Dismissing attachment does not stand

"I see no ships."

Lord Horatio Nelson, raising a telescope to his blind eye as the Danish Navy approached, Battle of Copenhagen, 1801

Denial can be defined as the conscious refusal to perceive that painful facts exist. By the use of denial, an individual can avoid intolerable thoughts, feelings or events. Groups and organisations, even governments, can also support denial. They can do this in their internal cultures, or as part of a wider cultural denial.

Working in two very large NHS trusts in England which provide specialist learning disability services to several counties, we have presented the issues as we see them in this book on several occasions to our colleagues. On one such occasion, a very senior clinician with an executive role responded to a talk given on trauma and attachment in the lives of people with intellectual disabilities, which included research evidence, with the comment, "You have no evidence for any of this".

Coming as this did from a person with great authority, with an international research profile, such a poorly informed opinion was very shocking to hear and prompted us to address this by seeking to engage in as many such talks as possible and was part of the motivation for writing this book.

The capacity for a person to deny information that contradicts their world view is well known (Bardon, 2020). Our esteemed colleague was a strong advocate of PBS, which has been the dominant model of clinical interventions since the 2000s and which incorporates Skinnerian conditioning (the impartial experimenter alters behaviour by either providing rewards or punishments to a target action by the 'subject') into an ethical system called *Social Role Valorisation*, which promotes 'adaptive' behaviours in place of 'challenging' behaviours.

In denying the undoubtable evidence that high rates of trauma and maltreatment are front, mid and centre to the problems of people with intellectual disability, this individual demonstrated *belief perseverance* (conceptual conservatism), which is the maintenance of a belief despite information that firmly contradicts it. Such beliefs can even be strengthened by evidence that contradicts the person's views. Humans are not essentially rational beings, but rather they are defensive, and do not seek to recognise cognitive dissonance, even (or *especially*?) if this would greatly benefit everyone concerned.

Nevertheless, we wanted to provide the evidence to undermine, hopefully fatally, the argument that current service philosophies and practices are somehow sufficient to prevent the maltreatment of people with intellectual disabilities, if only these could be done more diligently. We wanted to set forth such a clear argument for the importance of trauma-informed care and attachment-based interventions in intellectual disability services, that those who do not engage in flat denials will have the ammunition to remain constant in their conviction that change is necessary.

Childhood adversity and trauma is strongly predictive of physical and mental health outcomes

While adversity in childhood is not tantamount to trauma in childhood, it causes it directly and powerfully. Much research jumps from the adversity itself to the clinical outcomes in adulthood, notably the famous study by Felitti *et al* (1998). In brief, the Adverse Childhood Experiences study asked doctors in general practice in the West of the United States to routinely ask their patients if they had experienced any of ten common adversities. These were:

- Physical abuse.
- Sexual abuse or assault.
- Emotional belittling or verbal abuse.
- Being emotionally neglected.
- Witnessing domestic violence towards a parent.
- Lacking the basics of life such as food or shelter.
- Parental divorce or death.

- Parental mental health diagnosis.
- Imprisonment of a family member.
- Substance misuse in the family.

These experiences are common, and the rates of patients experiencing them were as follows – 0 ACEs, 33%; 1 ACE, 26%; 2 ACEs, 16%, 3 ACEs, 10%, 4 or more ACEs, 15%. The study found stark and strong associations between the number (multiplicity) of ACEs and the main public health priorities of modern societies – early smoking initiation, alcohol overuse, illicit drug use, obesity, suicide attempts, depression, anxiety, hallucination, teen and unwanted pregnancy, miscarriage, intimate partner violence, chronic obstructive pulmonary disease (COPD), Ischaemic heart disease, liver disease, lung cancer, and early death.

Figure 18.1: Mental health outcomes of adversity

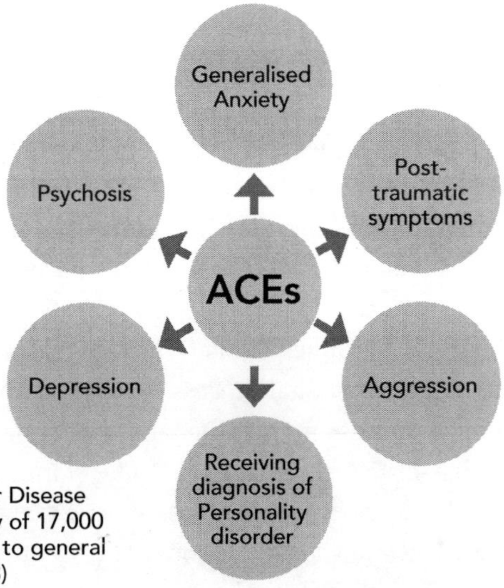

Source: Centre For Disease Control ACE Study of 17,000 people presenting to general practitioners (1998)

While in one sense it is helpful to have a direct understanding of the risks of ACEs to one's health, it is also important to consider how these events may actually traumatise a person, and how one's parents or caregivers can protect us from ACEs, or make their occurrence less damaging. An attachment relationship provides the freedom to explore, or 'play', because we are not worried about being safe. This requires us to have the kind of care as children that would provide this safety, as well as weaning us on guidance, from doing the thing together, to doing it under supervision, to being independent. However, it is often assumed that people value the skill or competency rather than the relationship with the caregiver itself, which supports this fun and learning. In fact, we contend that people are focused on forming, maintaining and seeking comfort from the relationships in their lives, and that tasks, activities and play are props to *enhance joyful, loving relationships*.

It should seem obvious to the reader that the ACEs listed above would entail the disturbance of the relationship between the child and the parent. For example, it would be very difficult to feel safe with a parent who sexually abuses you, punches you, or continually belittles you. A father who is physically abusing his spouse is unlikely to seem trustworthy to his children. Parents who are divorcing will be distracted at least some of the time from the care they would otherwise give their child. Imprisonment of a family member implies several potential risks, such as encouraged rule-breaking, economic desperation, absence of that person while in prison, etc. A lack of food and the basics of life demonstrates that a parent cannot or will not meet their children's needs to survive and/or thrive.

When we are securely attached, we can express emotions that are aversive to others without expecting to be silenced, attacked or rejected. This encourages us to recognise and think about our emotions, get on with others, deal with frustration, and not let bonds become ruptured in the face of difficulties. Our carers will be a model of safety, exploration, engagement and comforting at times of distress. We will internalise this and be able to use this emotional process with peers and others. We will experience more success in later life, and have a basic trust in others, rather than a basic suspicion. We will tend to form relationships that continue to provide a secure base and a safe haven, and our self-image will be positive. It will also be infectious. The security we offer in friendship and love will help those who have had less positive care experiences as children, because we will offer an alternative model – where their expectations are of intermittently available (e.g., ill, or addicted) parents, or hostile-dismissing parents who became aggressive to discourage the expression of emotions, we will disconfirm this. We may be perplexing to them, though.

When our parents could not or would not be consistently warm, competent and thoughtful about our feelings, we may worry that their state of mind will be variable. We may love them deeply and want to fix the problems they face. Perhaps we had to get our mother's medication for her, because she was too depressed to get out of bed. Perhaps our father had bouts of severe nausea from his chemotherapy treatment, which he did not want to worry us about, but he felt too sick to smile at us when we came to him. Perhaps one or both parents were struggling to overcome addiction, and overlooked our needs, then had terrible periods of guilt where they indulged us and were very kind. This leaves us worrying a lot about whether our peers or partners really like us; they find us unpredictable, even moody. Our self-esteem is unsure. We may need a considerable time in psychotherapy to unravel these processes, but eventually over time, through the secure attachments offered in therapy or by loving people in our lives, we can become essentially secure.

When our parents would respond to our approaches with anger or wanted us to be 'practical', perhaps saying, "I have not got time for you playing up", pushing us away, or fobbing us off on other family members, we may learn that emotions are to be avoided. We will not seek therapeutic help to talk about our emotions (because experience tells us that we will be hurt, rejected or belittled for doing so), but we might have other symptoms. It may be that we experience physical symptoms, sometimes frustrating our doctors by repeatedly turning up with seemingly real physical aches and pains that seem to have no underlying physical basis.

The psychoanalyst Adam Phillips remarked that trauma involves being captured by an event that cannot be experienced. By this he meant that something is too horrible to face *alone*. One of the principles of all forms of psychotherapy, even behavioural and cognitive therapies, is that we can think about the experience *together*. We would contend that there is a form of love required – a secure attachment – before the person can overcome trauma.

Attachment difficulties are linked to trauma and to outcomes

There is no scientific doubt of the link between child maltreatment and broken attachments on the one hand, and the outcomes of this maltreatment and relational damage on later physical and mental well-being. In a review of attachment theory as it affects people with intellectual disabilities, the British Psychological Society (2017) demonstrated that attachment difficulties in childhood were associated with:

- Difficulties in understanding the thoughts and feelings of others ('mentalising') as they enter school.
- Difficulties in getting on with other children when at primary school.
- Social anxiety and feeling incompetent with peers at secondary school.
- Receiving diagnoses of Attachment 'Disorder', 'Conduct Disorder' and 'Oppositional Defiant Disorder'.
- Being diagnosed with clinical anxiety.
- Being diagnosed with depression.
- Being diagnosed with obsessive-compulsive syndromes.
- Psychosis.
- Eating disorders.

These conditions represent the majority of the people who end up on the receiving end of mental health services, though the 'treatment' they receive, as we have shown in this book, can both reflect, and even re-enact, the way they have already been maltreated. To save costs, services are organised to have the smallest amount of personal contact that is required to keep a person from harming themselves or others. The emphasis is not on forming a personal relationship with the person as this is 'dependency' – which is little short of despised and reviled in service culture.

A colleague recently presented a service for people with 'personality disorders' in which they described the people they were trying to help by referring to them as 'Attachment-Seeking'. According to the practice of their service, this was to be avoided at all costs, and the recipients of the service were told in no certain terms that any lasting relationship with the team members was not on offer. We were horrified at the emotional rejection involved in such a stance (though the professionals were unaware of this). We saw this as a commonplace denial by health professionals in mental health services of the attachment needs of the oft-hurt, lonely and consistently rejected people whom they are charged to care for.

At the more extreme end of healthcare, some people just want to have a bed within a mental health setting. They need to go back before they can go forward. They will present with overdose, self-harming, standing on a bridge to communicate that they are considering jumping, etc., all to communicate the need for a healthier connection to a caring entity that will meet their needs.

Unfortunately, 'crisis' interventions are intended to check the current actual risk of them killing themselves, and then reduce this risk in the easiest/cheapest way for the system to achieve, and only in the short term. For those who experienced rejection or unavailable parents, this is confirmation that they are unworthy of care, pushing them back around their vicious circle of self-abuse and self-loathing. For those whose parents were unreliable, this just creates more and more anxiety, which takes a heavier and heavier toll on their minds, and they become intractably agitated and scan for kindness, somewhere, anywhere.

It is well known that the discharge of a patient from mental health services increases their risk of suicide (e.g., Chung *et al*, 2019). This fact alone and its lack of priority for government policy is an ongoing scandal, but should this be? A mental health ward offers food, company, warmth and a bed. There may be shouting, disturbances, restraints and even some violence, but there is a clear, basic form of care. Discharge – a word loaded with negative connotations of infection and unwantedness – marks the end of this care. Given that we are probably at our most vulnerable and needy at this time, it can be no surprise that the withdrawal of care in its intense, institutional form triggers earlier feelings of being unloved, unwanted. There may have been a lot of conflict at home, but at least there were 'three hots and a cot'.

Trauma is ubiquitous in the lives of people with intellectual disabilities

Global estimates of violence against children with disabilities, including intellectual disabilities, have recently been part of a worldwide meta-analytic study[39] that synthesised data from the English-speaking world and Chinese-speaking countries (Fang *et al*, 2022). The focus was on just under 100 studies that looked at the rate of maltreatment in a particular population.

The overall prevalence (recorded rate) of proven violence against children with disabilities was 31.7% (they estimated 95% likelihood that the true rate lies between 27.6% and 36.8%[40]) suggesting that the presence of a

39 A meta-analysis is a scientific paper which seeks to examine what the best-quality scientific papers designed to answer a question – in this case, if people with ID are more vulnerable to maltreatment – have found. They usually comment on the quality of evidence and what the evidence that is available can be concluded to show.

40 This is known as a 'confidence interval' which is helpful in that it gives a range which the true rate is likely to lie within, so that readers can see how much 'error' lays in the study results.

disability more than doubles the risk. Special statistical analyses indicated that the estimates were likely to be accurate, even though studies use different methods of study. The authors of the study noted that children with disabilities are burdened with the difficulties inherent in the disability as well as maltreatment, which is made worse by economic disadvantage.

However, we know that much abuse is not actually disclosed, so this is likely to be an underestimate.

These large-scale population studies are not designed to illustrate the individual and often tragic stories that people with intellectual disabilities experience. They say little about love, except by implication that phenomena like neglect and violence are not compatible with properly loving relationships. At a local level, we regularly find that almost all people with mild and moderate intellectual disabilities who see us for psychological therapy for problems like anxiety, depression, anger, over-checking behaviours, etc., will eventually disclose serious neglect and/or abuse in their childhoods. This can be incidentally found in research such as that testing the outcome of a particular psychotherapy. For example, Skelly *et al* (2018) found that 93% of people with mild and moderate intellectual disabilities offered psychodynamic therapy sessions were proved to have been sexually, physically, emotionally or financially abused, and usually more than one of these categories. In such sessions, not only does it become irrelevant if the person has limited language skills or needs help to live independently, but it also becomes very clear that they have never felt safe enough to disclose, never mind explain, their deep hurt. Given time, and by not imposing an agenda, as with more structured therapies, we have found that disclosures are more and more likely, sometimes after many months or even years of weekly sessions. Almost always, the recipient of the therapy will indicate some failure or rupture in their family of origin. They let us know that they have always felt somehow less than other people, that they have known all their lives and expect that no one is delighted just to be in their presence, and more often than not, that one or more other people saw them as a target for vitriol or exploitation.

It follows that in order to properly process and overcome such maltreatment, the person needs to be helped to think about their family of origin, and particularly their attachment to the person or persons who were charged with their early care.

Attachment is more often problematic in the lives of people with intellectual disabilities

A systematic review[41] of attachment in people with intellectual disabilities found clear evidence that people with intellectual disabilities are at higher risk of forming non-secure attachments to their carers (Hamadi & Fletcher, 2019). These findings were replicated in Canada, the Netherlands and Finland, suggesting that this may occur across Western cultures.

General interventions to address attachment

In the UK, around 80, 000 children were not living in their family of origin on 31st March 2022[42]. The Department for Education published figures of children in 2015/6 which recorded that over 32,000 children with Special Educational Needs (SEN) were either children 'in care' or at risk of going into care (the child is seen as 'in need' or in need of a *child protection plan*). While these figures are from two different years and some difference in the provision of care is expected, it should be clear that a sizeable proportion of children known to child protection services and who may be removed from their families of origin have intellectual disabilities.

The National Institute for Health and Care Excellence (NICE) published the Children's Attachment (NG26) in 2015 which was focused on the need for attachment-based interventions to prevent children who are known to the care system from having their life chances stunted by early maltreatment. Unfortunately, the guideline presents general guidelines for support and only mentions disability briefly, within the context of ensuring equality of access to attachment-based assessment and intervention, and without considering/ specifying adjustments to these interventions on the basis of the disability and how it affects the person's ability to form the close bonds that help overcome maltreatment. The evidence in the appendices does:

- insist that children with intellectual and other disabilities are in the scope of the guideline recommendations
- list 'learning disabilities' as a risk factor for attachment difficulties being worse when care is not adequate

41 A systematic review identifies, appraises and synthesises all available research relevant to a review question, in this case, whether intellectual disability is associated with an increased risk of Attachment difficulties.

42 Gov.UK website

- suggest that measuring intellectual disabilities may be assessed as part of an attachment-based assessment, as scientifically validated[43] tools are available.

The guideline does make striking recommendations that actually throw the care of adults with intellectual disabilities into sharp relief, especially the lack of any adult policy base based on attachment or other theories of emotional development, which we have mentioned elsewhere.

The guideline recommends:

- All children at risk of going into care, or in care, should have access to attachment-based interventions regardless of their social grouping (i.e. having an intellectual disabilities does not mean that attachment-based guidelines do not apply to you).
- The health, education and social care processes surrounding children should be stable and consistent, not fragmented and partial.
- All professional staff should be trained in attachment-based working, be able to screen for attachment difficulties, and know where the specialist services who can help are located. More specialist staff (social workers, post-care support, and others) should be able to form a measured opinion as to carer sensitivity, recognising the social and economic factors that affect outcomes, and know when to refer for evidence-based interventions.
- Video interaction guidance (VIG) should be available. VIG is an effective method of showing parents how they can improve recognising child distress, responding positively to expressions of feelings, behaving in ways that do not frighten children, and improving their own mastery of feelings that arise as they nurture their child.

Note that this is a specific Guideline from NICE that recommends the use of attachment theory to develop the whole system of care – as a core set of activities – to recognise distress, respond in helpful ways that promote emotional attunement, rather than using medication or conditioning (reward or punishment) to alter behaviours.

We believe that our current health and social care artificially ignores the attachment needs of people with intellectual disabilities, and that NICE

43 A tool that has been shown through scientific studies to be reliable (not containing too much 'error') and valid (measures what it says it measures).

NG26 is in fact highly relevant to the care system in which they live. There is, in fact, some research to back this up.

Specific interventions in specialist disability services

A specialist intervention was developed by Sterkenburg and colleagues in the Netherlands called Integrative Therapy for Attachment and Behaviour (ITAB). They reported a series of cases of children with multiple and complex disabilities, initially reported as a single case and then a case series, in order to address 'challenging behaviours' (Sterkenburg *et al*, 2008; Schuengel *et al*, 2009). The approach involves adding the development of an attachment relationship between therapist and child prior to engaging in a behavioural intervention. The authors suggest that the reinforcement from the positive relationship creates an advantageous set of 'contingencies' (mechanisms by which a person is encouraged to connect with others positively), allowing the child to experience more regulated emotions. In attachment terms, this means that an emotionally attuned adult can more successfully help a child with complex and multiple disabilities to feel less distressed, uncomfortable, and unstimulated. Importantly, the authors included a comparison control condition where the relationship was not developed prior to behavioural intervention, and where less positive change was observed.

Having helped the child directly, the therapist then moved to support daily caregivers to develop secure relationships with the child as well, before withdrawing. This approach is an explicit method of augmenting behavioural approaches, and the initial evidence suggests that it is an effective methodology that may be superior to behaviour modification provided by unfamiliar therapists. However, a study with more participants, random allocation to ITAB or control condition, and widening the approach to children without multiple disabilities, or adults with ID, would allow the findings to be generalised to other groups.

More recently, Vandesande *et al* (2022a) have developed an interview directly looking at the attachment strengths and needs of parents of children with severe/profound intellectual disabilities. Preliminary work on the scale shows that it has scientific acceptability and feasibility, suggesting it is useful to investigate further to check scientific validity. This follows other work by Vandesande *et al* (2022b) looking at how clinical professionals try to help parents connect with their children. There are also a range of tools available already for clinicians to assess attachment, which can be found in a document by the British Psychological Society (2017) entitled *Incorporating Attachment Theory into Practice*, which was the first document by that organisation to address attachment in people with intellectual disabilities.

People who have intellectual disabilities are often very articulate, where their disability has been described as 'mild' or 'moderate' (as opposed to 'severe' or 'profound'). There are a range of approaches to psychological therapies available in the UK which were summarised by the British Psychological Society in collaboration with the Royal College of Psychiatrists (2016). Of the different approaches available, Cognitive Analytic Therapy and Psychodynamic Psychotherapy are the most widely practised in terms of therapies that focus on relationships and how they are working or not working. Psychodynamic therapy in particular has been shown to improve outcomes for people referred for severe psychological distress. For example, Skelly *et al* (2018) measured the levels of psychological distress (as the person reported themselves) and general well-being as rated by a carer (a) on being referred in for help, (b) when assessed, (c) when the therapy was finished, and (d) at six-month follow up. They did not include people who received other interventions (a medication change, a behavioural therapy, an occupational therapist's input) so that as far as possible, any change would be likely to result from the therapy. They found that people did not improve significantly between being referred and being seen; they improved significantly and noticeably during the therapy; and this improvement was maintained when they were followed up. This supports and matches other studies by Beail *et al* (2005; 2007) who had found the same pattern of results in the clinic.

Now, this is not the gold-standard 'Randomised Controlled Trial' type of research, but it is good evidence that seeing a psychologist who properly listens to you about your distress, gets to know you, empathises, and stays available, is likely to coincide with a reduction in distress, and the earlier findings were *replicated* (the same finding was made by different researchers), which is telling us that such approaches are clearly onto something. Psychodynamic psychotherapy is well acquainted with thinking about love, hate, envy and other emotions, as well as being open to exploration of what happened in our family of origin, and what needs to happen to alleviate our distress, in terms of how we relate to others. We know from two important studies of this approach that clients themselves feel positive about their therapist and their therapy (Merriman & Beail,

2009), and that the great majority of people (indeed almost all) receiving this kind of therapy will rate that it made their life better, or a lot better (Khan & Beail, 2002).

We have already mentioned video feedback as a very effective way of improving attachment between a carer and a child with an intellectual disability. Damen *et al* (2011) developed the CONTACT intervention within group homes for children and adults with visual impairment and moderate to profound disability. In the system, professional caregivers refer a client whose relationship with them they consider to require improvement. The caregivers then review videotaped interactions with their client and are encouraged by a therapeutic coach to identify ways in which they could improve their relationship based largely on the principles of attachment theory. The study showed that the care staff became better at recognising and responding to the person's cues in ways that lowered their distress and promoted secure attachment behaviours. Not only this, but carers who may have shown signs that they might respond less helpfully to signs of distress in the client at the start of the intervention, had become more akin to secure caregivers by the end of the study. This study was completed with a relatively large number of carers (72) and this is again some good starting evidence that we can be as optimistic about developing security from insecure and disorganised Attachment in people with intellectual disabilities. A further study also found that this was associated with fewer reports of behaviours that carers consider challenging (van Wouwe, 2012).

These findings led the British Psychological Society (2017) to recommend that practitioners consider video feedback when supporting professional carers of people with severe intellectual disabilities.

Conclusions

Research is not equivocal in relation to the maltreatment of children, both in general and specifically with vulnerable groups of children, like those in care and those with intellectual disabilities, which overlap. The results are poorer outcomes in physical and psychological well-being. However, the need for awareness, enhanced help and specific interventions for children and adults with intellectual disabilities is not strong in the public consciousness or healthcare policy. The response of many clinicians, social care providers, policy advisers and governments is ambivalence. Something lurks behind 'least-needed' service protocols, reliance on brief clinical interventions even where these are not effective, underfunding and undervaluing of the heroic work of foster carers and others who seek long-term engagement, and the idea that mental health problems are the result of chemical or brain imbalances and defects, which might be amenable to drugs. Fear of 'dependency' is ubiquitous in our discourses on health and social care. It is as though offering a loving, long-term relationship to the loneliest and most often hurt people in our society will somehow deplete and bankrupt our society. People must learn to help themselves, even when this is beyond their ability to do so.

Our argument, based on our clinical experiences and the research available, is that:

- Childhood adversity and associated trauma vies to be the most powerful predictor of poor physical and mental health outcomes in adulthood.
- Promoting secure attachment in childhood and across the lifespan both prevents and ameliorates negative physical and mental health outcomes in adulthood.
- People with intellectual disabilities are exposed to heightened rates of childhood adversity and trauma, and even where these are not present, they experience micro-traumas in their everyday lives.
- Attachment is more likely to be disturbed in the childhoods of people with intellectual disabilities.
- The current emphasis on behavioural interventions within small but impersonal or even minimally staffed living placements is failing to meet the needs of people with intellectual disabilities, because their need for strong and enduring attachments to address limited emotional development, compounded by significant trauma in many cases, is not understood or valued, and is not mentioned in the current policy base.
- Attachment-based interventions are now being shown to be effective in addressing childhood trauma in children and adults with or without intellectual disabilities. Psychotherapy is effective in addressing complex trauma when the relationship with the therapist is strong, the person is allowed to freely explore, when they can engage for significant amounts of time, and when they perceive therapy as a safe space, a haven.
- Several research studies suggest that interventions that focus on relationships, either in psychotherapy for people with mild to moderate

intellectual disabilities, or in video interaction guidance for care teams of people with severe intellectual disabilities, are effective.

- No research exists that suggests that children with intellectual disabilities have any special resilience to maltreatment, therefore it is reasonable to assume that research demonstrating the detrimental effects of childhood trauma on physical and mental health has an urgent implication on their well-being, since maltreatment is visited upon them disproportionately.

In addition, there is no reason to expect that interventions for children in the care system based on attachment theory are not effective. It is often said that people with intellectual disabilities require a 'specific' evidence base; that is to say, we should not automatically expect treatments from the general population to work in people with intellectual disabilities – any proposed treatments need to have been shown to work on them – as a separately-studied group – before they are recommended.

We would challenge this view. Surely the onus is on those who would imply that people with intellectual disabilities do not benefit from relational interventions that are effective in people without disabilities to show that they do not work in that group? However, no such research is forthcoming, and the research that has been carried out almost always implies the opposite.

For example, Howard Steele et al (2019) published an excellent paper using the gold-standard research methodology for considering how effective attachment Interventions can be, the Randomised Controlled Trial or RCT[44]. In this study, they used Group Attachment-Based Intervention (GABI) with 43 families considered to be at risk of child maltreatment, versus 35 families receiving an established programme which included parent education in behavioural principles of not reinforcing difficult behaviours and encouraging desired behaviours (Systematic Training for Effective Parenting or STEP). This excellent research found that the families receiving the attachment-based interventions had markedly reduced levels of hostility, and reduced risk of child maltreatment to a

44 An RCT is a scientific trial of a new or existing treatment that involves *randomisation* to the treatment or a comparison group, where a clinician does not assess your suitability first; and *control*, which involves comparing any improvements in the treatment group a valid comparison group, such as people receiving an existing established treatment. In psychological interventions, a 'sham' or *placebo* is not possible, as one cannot be 'blinded' to the intervention one receives. However, it is possible to 'blind' the outcomes.

significantly greater extent than on the STEP programme. The parents themselves often had traumatic histories but benefitted as well.

There appears to be a widespread assumption that a child having a disability would somehow preclude such findings from applying to their health and social care.

We also wish to challenge the assumption that reducing challenging behaviours in and of themselves, or reducing 'symptoms' of mood disturbance, should be core outcomes for clinical services. Attachment theory explains how trauma can cause these to occur, but it should also provide the outcomes for services. Clinicians should be focused on achieving and maintaining significant, deep and enduring bonds in the lives of the people they work with. The feared 'placement breakdown' is, we would argue, more predictable from the level of fondness the carer feels for the person, than from the number of times they engage in a 'behaviour of concern'.

We know how to measure attachment bonds with psychometric tools, of course (BPS, 2017), but it is obvious in conversations with families, clients and care teams when they simply love the person at the centre of the care and would not be without them. Therefore, while we think about research, and are interested when it confirms or challenges our views, it is only one way of seeking knowledge. Reporting the emotional experience of people during counselling or carer support sessions is another, and through our direct contact with the people we have worked with, this has given us insights that research projects cannot. Or perhaps the very nature of research is that it is distanced and cannot notice a moment when love is beautifully confirmed in a smile or a touch, or when such moments are absent yet longed-for.

In one sense, the issue surrounds the policy base and its language. The UK's National Institute for Health and Care Excellence (NICE) has six sets of Guidance pertinent to people with intellectual disabilities at the time of writing (October, 2022). We have listed these with the total number of word search 'hits' for "Attachment" and "Trauma" below.

- *Social work with adults experiencing complex needs* (2022): Attachment – 0, Trauma – 0
- *Disabled children and young people up to 25 with severe complex needs: integrated service delivery and organisation across health, social care and education* (2022): Attachment – 0, Trauma – 0

- *Care and support of people growing older with learning disabilities*: Attachment – 0, Trauma – 0.
- *Learning disabilities and behaviour that challenges: service design and delivery* (2018): Attachment – 0, Trauma – 0.
- *Mental health problems in people with learning disabilities: prevention, assessment and management* (2014): Attachment – 0, Trauma – 1 (a mild piece of advice for professionals to understand that "psychological factors [such as trauma]" (p.43) could cause mental health problems).
- *Challenging behaviour and learning disabilities: prevention and interventions for people with learning disabilities whose behaviour challenges* (2015): Attachment – 0, Trauma – 1 (one bullet point, indicating that trauma should be noted during assessment).

Those writing the guidelines do not ask the right questions about the emotional and relationship histories of people with intellectual disabilities. There has been no *Guideline Development Group* formed to address the scandalously high levels of abuse and neglect of people with intellectual disabilities, though surely this should be a clear priority. There has been no *Guideline Development Group* formed to address the high rates of disturbed attachment.

Who asks people with learning disabilities if they have enough love in their life? Many researchers have looked at sexual knowledge and opportunities for sexual relations, seeing this as wanting. Murphy and O'Callaghan (2004) demonstrated that adults with intellectual disabilities had significantly less formal knowledge about most aspects of sex and appeared more vulnerable to abuse. These authors suggested that many of the adults with intellectual disabilities had trouble distinguishing abusive and consenting relationships. While this study was largely based on line-drawings and formal questioning (rather than examples from their real lives), the authors suggested that what was needed was ongoing access to sex education.

Surely, though, we need safety, guidance, companionship and comfort, long before we need sexual interactions. We also know that sexual partners will be picked on the basis of our attachment history (e.g., Frazier *et al*, 2005), not even within our conscious knowledge or awareness, which helps to explain why attachment problems pass through the generations. Given the huge rate at which people with intellectual disabilities are maltreated in all its various forms, some or even most of the lack of 'sexual knowledge' that they demonstrate could reflect the lack of emotional security in their childhood. This would not necessarily respond to formal education, because attachment patterns do not follow one's formal understanding of sex, consent etc., but rather meet the need to match the earlier template provided by the early care relationship.

While not suggesting that research into sexual knowledge is unhelpful, this emphasis on comparing abilities based on chronologically age-matched groups to people with intellectual disabilities makes an *a priori* assumption that they will have the same starting point in life. They do not. People with intellectual disabilities are more likely to be traumatised by adversity, and more likely to have multiple adversities as children and afterwards. They are more likely to come from families with lower incomes, and they are more likely to have attachment problems, be taken into the care system, and be exposed to non-family-style care, which is often institutional and poorly attuned to their emotional needs. Any expectation that most people with intellectual disabilities will achieve appropriate levels of knowledge to keep themselves safe and successfully negotiate relationships, with these differences in mind, must be naïve, to say the least.

That is to say, if we have not been properly loved as children, or not loved at all, we should not be expected to be able to achieve satisfying, loving relationships as adults, or even know where to begin. We will simply act according to the life we have known.

The gap between the evidence and any awareness by policymakers that something radical needs to happen is at once obvious, alarming, and urgent. Yet the myopia of bodies like NICE is remarkable. There can be no policy base to address what we have described in this book until the research is translated into a proper policy base that will truly address the need for people with intellectual disabilities by providing the concepts, evidence and actions required to provide family-style care based on attachment principles, while acknowledging the ubiquity of trauma. One might even go as far as Sinason (2021) and say that "the history of intellectual disability is a history of trauma".

We set forth our views on what is required in the final short chapter of this book.

References

Bardon A (2020) Coronavirus responses highlight how humans are hardwired to dismiss facts that don't fit their worldview. *The Conversation Online*, 127168.

British Psychological Society (2017) *Incorporating Attachment Theory into Practice: Clinical Practice Guideline for Clinical Psychologists working with People who have Intellectual Disabilities.* Leicester, UK: British Psychological Society.

Chung D, Hadzi-Pavlovic D, Wang M *et al* (2019) Meta-analysis of suicide rates in the first week and the first month after psychiatric hospitalisation. *British Medical Journal Open*, 9: e023883. doi: 10.1136/bmjopen-2018-023883

Damen S, Kef S, Worm M, Janssen MJ & Schuengel C (2011) Effects of video-feedback interaction training for professional caregivers of children and adults with visual and intellectual disabilities. *Journal of Intellectual Disability Research* **55** 581–595.

Fang F, Cerna-Turoff I, Zhang C, Lu M, Lachman JM & Barlow J (2022) Global estimates of violence against children with disabilities: an updated systematic review and meta-analysis. *The Lancet Child & Adolescent Mental Health.* doi: 10.1016/S2352-4642(22)00033-5

Felitti VJ, Anda RF, Nordenberg D, Williamson DF, Spitz AM *et al* (1998)Relationship of childhood abuse and household dysfunction to many of the leading causesof death inadults: The Adverse Childhood Experiences (ACE) Study. *American Journal of Preventative Medicine* **14** 245–258.

Frazier P, Byer A, Fischer A, Wright D & Debord K (2005) Adult attachment style and partner choice: Correlational and experimental findings. *Personal Relationships* **3** 117.

Hamadi L & Fletcher HK (2019) Are people with an intellectual disability at increased risk of attachment difficulties? A critical review. *Journal of Intellectual Disabilities* **25** (1) 114-130.

National Institute for Health and Clinical Excellence (NICE NG26; 2015) *Children's Attachment: Attachment in children and young people who are adopted from care, in care or at high risk of going into care* [online]. Available at nice.org.uk

Schuengel C, Sterkenburg PS, Jeczynski P, Janssen CGC & Jongbloed G (2009) Supporting affect regulation in children with multiple disabilities during psychotherapy: a multiple case design study of therapeutic attachment. *Journal of Consulting and Clinical Psychology* **77** 291–301.

Sinason V (2021) The history of disability is a history of trauma. In Frankish, P., Beail, N. & Skelly, A. (eds) *Trauma and Intellectual Disability: Acknowledgement, Identification and Intervention.* West Sussex: Pavilion Publishing.

Skelly A, McGeehan C & Usher R (2018) An open trial of psychodynamic psychotherapy for people with mild-moderate intellectual disabilities with waiting list and follow up control. *Advances in Mental Health and Intellectual Disabilities* **12** (5/6) 153–162.

Steele H, Murphy A, Bonuck K, Meissner P & Steele M (2019) Randomized control trial report on the effectiveness of Group Attachment-Based Intervention (GABI©): Improvements in the parent-child relationship not seen in the control group. *Development and Psychopathology* **31** (1) 203–217.

Sterkenburg PS, Janssen CGC & Schuengel C (2008) The effect of an attachment-based behaviour therapy for children with visual and severe intellectual disabilities. *Journal of Applied Research in Intellectual Disabilities* **21** 126–135.

Vandesande S, Bosmans G, Sterkenburg P, Schuengel C & Maes B (2022) The Attachment Strengths and Needs Interview for parents of children with severe or profound intellectual disabilities: An acceptability and feasibility study, *Journal of Intellectual & Developmental Disability* **47** (2) 118-130.

Van Wouwe H (2012) Triple C: researching the effects of treatment. *Journal of Intellectual Disability Research* **56** 683–683.

Chapter 19: Putting love at the heart of care services

"Children who have experienced neglect, abuse, exploitation, torture or who are victims of war must receive special support to help them recover their health, dignity, self-respect and social life."

Article 39, UN Declaration on the Rights of the Child

"I think everyone needs love. No one wants to be without any friends or family or a boyfriend. Everyone should have someone."

Person with an intellectual disability, cited in Matilla *et al*, 2017

If you have read this far you will not be surprised by our views on how health and social care should be organised for people with intellectual disabilities. The onus is on care services to do the following:

1. Acknowledge that people with intellectual disabilities have a 'double whammy' of cognitive difficulties and raised exposure to adversity and trauma.
2. Acknowledge that many people are not emotionally developed enough, or have experienced too much trauma, to share their carer with others or live in groups.
3. Organise services to have relational goals rather than reductions in mental health symptoms or 'eliminating challenging behaviours'.
4. Related to point 3, to alter the narrative of policies aimed at people with intellectual disabilities and build policy within the language of attachment and not the language of mental health illness, risk assessment, behaviourism, or, worst of all, economics.
5. Recognising that, for many, focusing on controlling their distress or challenging behaviours is oppressive, while at the same time, their trauma histories are ignored. Thus, many healthcare interventions are re-traumatising and there are many instances of sadistic care that keep recurring throughout history.

6. Such scandals only come to light through undercover work by the media, and not through organisational safeguarding procedures and organisations like to Care Quality Commission (CQC) who did not act when approached by whistleblower Terry Bryan about abuse at Winterbourne View Hospital in 2011[45], and gave Newbus Grange Hospital an 'outstanding' rating just five months before rating it as 'inadequate'[46]; the latter inspection only occurring after the BBC's Panorama had uncovered serious abuse at the notorious Whorlton Hall[47].
7. This illustrates that only close observation really reveals the truth about the care of people who either lack the language skills to report on their care, or whose opinions are not valued enough for them to have a strong voice.

Care should be:

- Intimate.
- Small scale, with a family feel.
- Unconditional.
- Fun and delight-full.
- Enjoyable for everyone.
- An Onion Skin of Care, where the carers feel cared for.
- Focused on safety.
- Focused on exploration and learning.
- Focused on staying engaged.
- Based on relational goals and not symptom reduction or behaviour change.
- Less focused on mental 'illness' as a source of distress.
- Mindful of trauma, relationship losses and failures of past care.
- Not defined by 'challenging behaviours'.
- Less focused on 'independence skills' purely to reduce reliance on care relationships.

---

45 *Winterbourne View 'failed to protect people'.* BBC News, 18th July 2011. The CQC claimed in their own report that Mr Bryan's complaints to them did not contain the allegations later uncovered by an undercover BBC investigation. However, Mr Bryan stated that he had approached the BBC because of the lack of action from the company management and the CQC.

46 *Darlington & Stockton Times*, 25th September 2019.

47 *Undercover Hospital Abuse Scandal.* BBC One, 22nd May 2019.

In short, a loving, family-style situation with minimal exposure to childhood adversity should be seen as a basic right, and even more of a priority for children (and many if not most adults) with intellectual disabilities, who have endured myopia, injustice, callousness, hardship, unacknowledged losses, and even hate crimes, for far too long.

Policy, practice, care service commissioning, and professionals working in the field should set up services to provide deep and enduring attachments for people with intellectual disabilities. Their words and behaviours can be understood within the guiding ideas of attachment theory, to help determine exactly what they need. Financial and resource barriers are only part of the problem here. We argue that the values base of intellectual disabilities services is misconceived, focusing on the attainment of adult rights, financial independence and employment, none of which address the central problem of being expected to function emotionally way beyond the level that one's emotional development can support. Further, the medicalisation of human distress and the continuing influence of Skinnerian Behaviourism create the illusion that the high rates of so-called mental ill-health in people with intellectual disabilities can be addressed by medication, behavioural programmes, or skills teaching programmes. Between us, we have more than 40 years' experience of these attempts within community care services in the UK, and we can attest their overall effect on the lives of people with intellectual disabilities is risible. Despite their panacea promise, psychiatry and behavioural psychology have failed to stop repeated scandals and, increasingly, we feel that they are part of the problem, containing as they do unfulfilled promises of liberation and positive change.

What should be done instead?

Where there has been emotional neglect (as with Lesley, Renata and Leonard), there should be a relentless focus on personal connection and the formation of, or improvement in, significant attachments. These attachments need to be emotionally attuned and oriented to the person's level of emotional development.

Where a person is described as 'attention seeking' (as with Leonard, LeBron and Lucy), attachments should be strengthened, not diminished or denied.

Where a person demonstrates 'sensory behaviours' (as with LeBron, Murray and Leonard), this should not negate their need for attachment, and it should be considered that they might be soothing themselves in the absence of an emotionally attuned Significant Other. It should never be accepted that a person is 'asocial'.

Where a person is seen as 'difficult' or 'non-compliant' (as with Colin, Lesley, LeBron and Lucy), this is likely to have something to do with their emotional development and may to a large degree be a matter of *acceptance* in relation to their level of functioning, following the stage model. We should not try to 'condition' their attempts to control their environment out of existence unless this is consistent with their level of emotional functioning. Compliance – never challenging others – is not desirable in and of itself.

Where a person with an intellectual disability has been abused or neglected (every case described in this book, as well as many, many other people), there should be public acknowledgement and solemn atonement. A trauma-informed understanding of each person's life should be incorporated into their medical and care records, so that future responses to stress will have the correct context and not be seen as 'abnormal'. This works against medical models that imply that chemical imbalances are causal of mental illnesses that are observed in 'challenging behaviours', and that require the primary use of medications, which did such terrible damage to the life of Jennifer. We see only a very limited future for medication in alleviating the suffering of people with intellectual disabilities when what they are really missing is love.

We see no future in any form for institutional care. These places cannot provide love. The use of the term 'care' regarding their continuation should stick in all our throats. It will only be when all bonds of care are felt to be as strong as they are for a member of one's family that resilience will truly appear in health and social care services.

"As special needs parents, we don't have the power to make the world 'fair', but we do have the power to make it joyful."

Anonymous

"Children with disabilities need a little more. Don't push a little one away when they're naughty or ask for attention. That's how we get mental health problems; because we think: 'No one loves me'."

Roger Wilczek, expert by experience, 2021

References

Mattila J, Määttä K & Uusiautti S (2017) 'Everyone needs love' –an interview study about perceptions of love in people with intellectual disability (ID). *International Journal of Adolescence and Youth* **22** (3) 296-307.

Wilczek R (2021) Please stop people going through what I went through – and am still going through. In: Beail, N., Frankish, P. & Skelly, A. (eds) *Trauma and Intellectual Disability: Acknowledgment, Identification and Intervention.* Shoreham, West Sussex: Pavilion Publishing.